QBASE ANAESTHESIA: 1
MCQs FOR THE ANAESTHESIA PRIMARY

QBASE ANAESTHESIA: 1
MCQs FOR THE ANAESTHESIA PRIMARY

Edited by

Edward Hammond MA BM BCh MRCP FRCA
Shackleton Department of Anaesthetics
Southampton University Hospital NHS Trust

Andrew McIndoe MB ChB FRCA
Sir Humphrey Davy Department of Anaesthetics
Bristol Royal Infirmary

Authors
Mark Blunt
Andrew Cone
Edward Hammond
John Isaac
Andrew McIndoe
Andrew Scott
John Urquhart

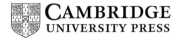

CAMBRIDGE
UNIVERSITY PRESS

CAMBRIDGE UNIVERSITY PRESS
Cambridge, New York, Melbourne, Madrid, Cape Town, Singapore, São Paulo

Cambridge University Press
The Edinburgh Building, Cambridge, CB2 8RU, UK

Published in the United States of America by Cambridge University Press, New York

www.cambridge.org
Information on this title: www.cambridge.org/9780521687980

First published 1997
Reprinted 1998
Reprinted by Cambridge University Press 2007

Printed in the United Kingdom at the University Press, Cambridge

A catalogue record for this book is available from the British Library

ISBN-13 978-0-521-68798-0 paperback

CONTENTS

QBase Anaesthesia on CD-ROM

FOREWORD

One useful piece of advice for candidates for any examination is to remind them that it is better to make any mistakes at home rather than in the examination room. It is also cheaper. Examination technique needs practice.

Multiple choice examinations are a common feature of most postgraduate medical examinations. They are easier to mark than essays. They should remove the element of examiner bias which can (although rarely) cloud the judgement of essays and oral examinations. MCQs also seek to establish the knowledge of the 'facts' of a subject. Occasionally one year's facts become next year's myths. I remember too well that in my under graduate days there were 48 chromosomes in a man: somehow we have come down to 46. But at least the 'correct' facts are the same for every candidate.

The Royal College of Anaesthetists has used MCQs for many years in its examinations. The revised Primary FRCA examination uses a large bank of questions and the new paper will have 90 questions each with five parts. The balance will be approximately 30 in pharmacology, 30 in physiology and biochemistry, 15 in physics and clinical measurement, 10 in clinical anaesthesia and 5 in statistics. The paper takes three hours, giving some two minutes for each question. Candidates will need to avoid wasting time and have a good technique.

Hammond and McIndoe have produced this CD as an interactive guide to the examination using a bank of questions covering the areas described in the College syllabus. Those using it can opt for a full paper made up in the college format or a defined, but random selection. The bank is comprehensive although not as large as the College's one. There are two useful additions which will help the learning process. Firstly, in addition to giving the correct answers, the questions are annotated indicating some of the thinking behind the question and also give some useful external references. The second feature is as important. When trying out the answers, we can indicate whether we feel certain of the answer, whether we have made an educated guess or whether we have just made a guess. In the ensuing analysis, we will learn whether our guesses are as educated as we think they are and also of the danger of making uneducated guesses. Candidates for MCQ exams need to realise the penalties in making guesses: the result is likely to be a reduction in mark, not an improvement. By trying out the programs on this disk, candidates should learn to avoid that fatal error.

I could hope that the College might be persuaded to publish its question bank. Everyone might then learn the correct answers and gain 100% on the mark. That ought to be the acceptable standard. MCQs, if they test facts, should be marked as a pass-fail examination and not as a ranking examination. This CD is an excellent guide to the new Primary: those who use it intelligently will check their knowledge, perhaps learn some more and most importantly, learn how to cope with this type of examination.

JOHN NORMAN
Professor of Anaesthetics
the University of Southampton

INTRODUCTION

"2B or not 2B. That is the question.
To guess or not to guess. That is the problem"

Q*Base Anaesthesia* has been designed to help you improve your exam technique and maximise your chance of passing the Primary FRCA.

The new Primary FRCA examination encompassed much of the knowledge previously required for the old Part I and II examination. Reading through the new syllabus can be a daunting experience for those of us who have passed the old style exams. The multiple choice examination for the Primary FRCA is made up of 90 questions; 30 Physiology, 30 Pharmacology, 15 Equipment/Physics/Measurement, 10 Clinical Anaesthesia and 5 Statistics. The time allowed is three hours.

The negative marking system for the multiple choice exam can leave a bitter taste in the mouth of the candidate. There is no substitute for knowledge, revision and adequate preparation for the exam. Exam technique is an important part of the preparatory process. No ones knowledge is complete. Tutors differ in the advice they give on whether candidates should guess. Some advise that candidates should guess and answer all the questions. Others advise that candidates should only answer those they are sure of. Between these black and white pieces of advice, there remains every shade of grey.

The questions in the book include referenced notes and explanations. The questions have been designed to cover as much of the new Primary syllabus as possible. Some are harder than others. Some may seem impossible whereas others may be straight forward. They are designed to test the candidate but also to educate. The comprehensive referenced notes aim to improve your knowledge and point you in the right direction for further reading. The book is arranged into 5 papers of 90 questions and follows the format of the actual exam.

BUT THIS IS NOT JUST ANOTHER MCQ BOOK

This book comes with a Interactive CD-ROM containing the **QBase Interactive MCQ Examination System**. The CD-ROM contains 50 questions more than the book. For the novice user there is a quick start option with the same 5 papers as in the book presented as as interactive on screen examination.

The CD-ROM has many advantages over the book. It allows candidates to build a customised exam for themselves. The candidate may select a mock exam of 90 questions chosen from the 500 questions or a customised exam containing any number of questions from any number of the 5 main topics in the Primary Exam. The emphasis is on choice. The CD-ROM includes automated marking and results analysis as well as the option to store the exam with your answers for a later review. The exam can also be repeated with the leaves to each question shuffled which eliminates the element of pattern recognition that can falsely elevate a candidates score. Furthermore the CD-ROM includes the

Confidence Level Option which allows the candidate to tag his level of certainty to an answer for later analysis. This option allows the candidate to analyse the effect of his guessing strategy on his final score for the exam.

QBase Anaesthesia on CD-ROM has been designed to be easy to use. No knowledge of computers is necessary. It encompasses the experience of many of us who have sat negatively marked MCQ exams and have tried to determine what the best answering technique should be. The program will help you improve your exam techniques and maximise your score. We hope you will find it a useful tool in your preparation for the Primary FRCA examination.

EDWARD HAMMOND
ANDREW MCINDOE
Southampton and Bristol

ACKNOWLEDGMENTS

We would like to thank Asif Choudhory for his help in programming the system, Derek Virtue for reverse engineering the book from the CD-ROM, Lucy Gardner for copy editing the manuscript in electronic format, the publisher, Geoff Nuttall and Drs David Wilkins, Brian Sweeney and Maher Michel for their support and encouragement.

Exam 1

QUESTION 1

The following can be found in normal adult venous blood

A. 3% COHb
B. 5% MetHb
C. 70% OxyHb
D. 2% free Hb
E. 2% HbA_2

QUESTION 2

The following are true of humidifiers

A. A heat-moisture exchanger (HME) is more efficient than a cold water bath with gas bubbled through.
B. A heated bath can provide humidification greater than that seen in the normal upper trachea.
C. A cold water bath can provide humidification greater than that seen in the normal upper trachea.
D. An ultrasonic nebulizer can provide a relative humidity of 200% at 37°C
E. Normal humidity in the upper trachea is 440 g/m^3.

QUESTION 3

Opioid receptors

A. Can currently be classified as mu, delta, kappa and sigma.
B. All mediate analgesia.
C. When activated cause an increase in neurotransmitter release.
D. May be found in the knee joint.
E. Possess their own endogenous ligands.

QUESTION 4

The following drugs can cause significant histamine release

A. Pancuronium.
B. Amitryptilline.
C. Suxamethonium.
D. Pethidine.
E. Ketamine.

QUESTION 5

Cardiac output increases with

A. An increase in stroke volume.
B. An increase in dp/dt.
C. An increase in LVEDV.
D. An increase in pulmonary venous pressure.
E. An increase in aortic pressure.

QUESTION 6

The following adversely affect the outcome of ventricular defibrillation

A. Increasing time from onset of ventricular fibrillation (VF) to first defibrillation.
B. An initial rhythm at time of defibrillation of ventricular fibrillation as opposed to asystole.
C. Acidosis.
D. Defibrillation during inspiration.
E. Digoxin toxicity.

QUESTION 7

With regard to magnesium

A. It is the second most plentiful cation in the body.
B. Approximately 1% is in the extracellular compartment.
C. Approximately 25% is in bone.
D. Aldosterone increases its renal excretion.
E. Parathyroid hormone (PTH) enhances the absorption from the gut.

QUESTION 8

Confidence intervals

A. Indicate the presence or otherwise of a statistical difference between groups.
B. Are large if the sample size is small.
C. A 95% confidence interval means that 95% of all observed values fall within that interval.
D. When considering an odds ratio, if the 95% confidence interval includes unity then no significant difference may apply.
E. The confidence interval gives a range of values within which the true value will lie.

QUESTION 9

Regarding the renal circulation

A. A renal blood flow of 1200 ml/min is likely if the mean arterial presure is 160 mmHg.
B. Blood supply to the medulla is derived entirely from the vasa recta.
C. Macula densa cells are located in the afferent arteriolar wall.
D. Autoregulation of renal blood flow occurs in the denervated kidney.
E. Renal oxygen consumption is approximately 60 ml/min.

QUESTION 10

Insulin exerts its hormonal effect in target cells

A. By inducing changes in enzyme configuration.
B. By altering the rate of enzyme synthesis.
C. By altering substrate availability.
D. Following intracellular phosphorylation of a membrane receptor.
E. Following conjugation with a 33 amino acid C-chain.

QUESTION 11

Steroid hormones

A. May all be derived from cholesterol.
B. Can be synthesized by the placenta.
C. Which are classed androgens have 18 C atoms.
D. May all be derived from progesterone.
E. Hydroxylated at C atom 21 are all mineralocorticoids.

QUESTION 12

Non-parametric tests

A. Can be used on small samples.
B. Can be used to analyse samples that are normally distributed.
C. Include Student's paired t-test.
D. Can be applied to ordinal data.
E. Should not be used if the nature of the distribution of the data is unknown

QUESTION 13

Activity of the gastric parietal cells

A. Includes ATP driven exchange of sodium ions for hydrogen ions.
B. Can give rise to secretions of pH 1.0.
C. Includes release of gastrin.
D. Requires the presence of carbonic anhydrase.
E. Is stimulated by hypoglycaemia.

QUESTION 14

The following drugs have active metabolites

A. Suxamethonium.
B. Captopril.
C. Codeine.
D. Propranolol.
E. Phenobarbitone.

QUESTION 15

Regarding the smoking of tobacco

- **A.** Smoking is associated with oxyhaemoglobin desaturation in recovery in children of smokers.
- **B.** Carboxyhaemoglobin may be distinguished from oxyhaemoglobin by pulse oximetry.
- **C.** A carboxyhaemoglobin level of 15% will reduce the maximal haemoglobin saturation to 85% on room air.
- **D.** Abstinence from smoking for 12 hours restores airway sensitivity to that of the non-smoker.
- **E.** Smoking is associated with an increased incidence of diabetes mellitus.

QUESTION 16

Compensation to acute haemorrhage includes

- **A.** Increased baroreceptor stretch.
- **B.** Cerebral vasoconstriction.
- **C.** Renal efferent arteriolar vasoconstriction.
- **D.** Increased circulating angiotensin II.
- **E.** Reduced chemoreceptor discharge.

QUESTION 17

The following agents are bacteriostatic

- **A.** Sulphadimidine.
- **B.** Chloramphenicol.
- **C.** Rifampicin.
- **D.** Tetracyclines.
- **E.** Fucidic acid.

QUESTION 18

The heat–moisture exchanger (HME)

- **A.** Is more effective at higher tidal volumes.
- **B.** Contains a mesh on which exhaled humidity can condense.
- **C.** May be bactericidal.
- **D.** Performance is consistent for 24 hour.
- **E.** Can help prevent passage of viral particles.

QUESTION 19

Chronic airways disease.

A. Dyspnoea at rest and a PaO_2 < 7.2 predict the need for postoperative ventilatory support.
B. Cor pulmonale is associated with a raised JVP and left ventricular failure.
C. FEV_1 <1 litre is an absolute contraindication to general anaesthesia.
D. Postoperative respiratory depression is most pronounced on the second and third postoperative nights.
E. Sedative premedication with pulse oximetry is appropriate.

QUESTION 20

Diamorphine.

A. Is a naturally occurring opioid.
B. Crosses the blood-brain barrier where it is an agonist at mu opioid receptors.
C. Is rapidly hydrolysed to inactive metabolites.
D. Has a greater potential for physical dependence than morphine.
E. Is poorly lipid soluble.

QUESTION 21

If the rate of transfer of a drug is defined as change in concentration divided by time (dC/dT)

A. dC/dT is constant for a first order process.
B. dC/dT = -k.C for a zero order process.
C. A plot of concentration against time will produce a hyperbola.
D. Integration of the equation reveals the volume of distribution.
E. Passive drug transfer is almost always first order.

QUESTION 22

The use of inhaled nitric oxide in ARDS

A. Decreases systemic arterial pressure.
B. Decreases pulmonary arterial pressure.
C. Increases intrapulmonary shunt.
D. Leads to toxic side effects in inspired concentrations of 1-10 ppm.
E. Improves arterial oxygen tension.

QUESTION 23

Cardiac ventricular muscle

A. Repolarization time varies with cardiac rate.
B. Depolarization is followed by a plateau potential lasting about 200 ms.
C. Prepotential decay between action potentials is due to declining K^+ efflux.
D. Cannot be tetanized.
E. Action potential amplitude is dependent on extracellular Na concentration.

QUESTION 24

In the heart

  A. Depolarization takes place from epi- to endocardium.
  B. Depolarization takes place from the apex of the ventricles to the base.
  C. Speed of conduction of excitation is termed chronotropy.
  D. Excitability via alteration in pacemaker cell threshold potential is termed bathmotropy.
  E. Contractility of the myocardium is termed inotropy.

QUESTION 25

During nocturnal sleep

  A. Periods of rapid eye movement are accompanied by 3 Hz spikes and waves on the EEG.
  B. Dreams tend to occur during periods of rapid eye movement.
  C. Delta waves on the EEG are associated with deep sleep.
  D. Core temperature typically drops half a degree Celsius.
  E. ACTH plasma levels fall until approximately 6am.

QUESTION 26

The following drugs exhibit tachyphylaxis

  A. Glyceryl trinitrate.
  B. Ephedrine.
  C. Succinylcholine.
  D. Trimetaphan.
  E. Hydralazine.

QUESTION 27

The MAC (minimum alveolar concentration) is reduced in the following situations.

  A. Hypothermia.
  B. Female sex.
  C. Chronic alcoholism.
  D. Prolonged duration of anaesthesia.
  E. Hypothyroidism.

QUESTION 28

Comparing alfentanil with fentanyl

  A. Fentanyl has a lower potency.
  B. Fentanyl is more ionized at pH 7.4.
  C. Fentanyl has a larger volume of distribution.
  D. Fentanyl has a higher clearance.
  E. Fentanyl is more extensively protein bound.

QUESTION 29

During fat absorption and metabolism

A. Naturally occuring fatty acids contain an odd number of carbon atoms.
B. Free fatty acids remain unbound to albumin.
C. Chylomicrons are broken down to triglycerides by lipoprotein lipase.
D. Low density lipoproteins are broken down into very low density lipoproteins and have a role as cholesterol carriers.
E. Beta-oxidation involves serial cleaving of 1- carbon fragments from the fatty acid molecule.

QUESTION 30

The following are true

A. Decontamination implies the removal or killing of most or all infective organisms.
B. Gamma irradiation is convenient for sterilisation in theatres.
C. HIV is highly resistant to hypochlorite solutions.
D. Electrically-powered ventilators should be disinfected with alcohol rather than aqueous solutions.
E. Gluteraldehyde can be used for disinfection and sterilisation.

QUESTION 31

Regarding day surgery

A. Insulin-dependant patients may be considered if starved overnight.
B. Gastro-oesphageal reflux is not a contraindication to day surgery.
C. The patient may not drive nor operate machinery for 24 hours post operatively but preparing hot food is acceptable.
D. Regional anaesthesia is contraindicated.
E. Suxamethonium apnoea and malignant hyperpyrexia are contraindications to day surgery.

QUESTION 32

Esmolol

A. Is useful in the treatment of essential hypertension.
B. Has a half life of ten minutes.
C. Is rapidly metabolised by the liver.
D. Acts selectively on beta-1 receptors.
E. Possesses intrinsic sympathomimetic activity.

QUESTION 33

The Venturi principle may be used in

A. Fixed performance oxygen masks ('Ventimask').
B. Humidification.
C. Suction apparatus.
D. Scavenging.
E. Ventilation.

QUESTION 34

Methohexitone

A. Is a sulphated oxybarbiturate.
B. In solution has a pH of 8.2.
C. Has an elimation half-life of 3 hours.
D. Tends to cause excitatory phenomenaon induction.
E. Has been used as an anticonvulsant.

QUESTION 35

Consequences of intermittent positive pressure ventilation (IPPV) include

A. Diuresis.
B. Increased cerebral perfusion pressure.
C. Decreased functional residual capacity.
D. Decreased cardiac output.
E. Increased dead space.

QUESTION 36

Obesity is associated with

A. An increase in the incidence of airway complications.
B. Increased functional residual capacity (FRC).
C. Increased DO_2 (Oxygen delivery).
D. Pulmonary hypertension.
E. Quetelet index of 24.5.

QUESTION 37

The following occur at 36 weeks of pregnancy

A. Reduced FRC.
B. Increased residual volume.
C. Increased tidal volume.
D. Increased $PaCO_2$.
E. Increased renal bicarbonate loss.

QUESTION 38

Latent heat of vaporisation

A. Is the energy required to change a liquid to vapour at a constant temperature.

B. Increases as the temperature increases.

C. Is infinite at the critical temperature.

D. Is the principle behind a form of anaesthesia.

E. It may cause inaccuracies in vaporisers.

QUESTION 39

The following actions are known prostaglandin effects

A. Bronchial muscle relaxation.

B. Inhibition of gastrointestinal secretion.

C. Uterine relaxation.

D. Bronchial muscle contraction.

E. Fever.

QUESTION 40

Warfarin

A. Is a member of the inanedione family.

B. Inhibits the synthesis of prothrombin only.

C. Is well absorbed.

D. Is 95% bound to the globulin fraction.

E. Is contraindicated in early pregnancy.

QUESTION 41

Measuring cardiac output by the thermodilution method

A. Injecting less than the required volume of injectate leads to an over-estimation of the cardiac output.

B. Injection should be performed over about ten seconds.

C. Looping of the catheter in the right ventricle may cause inaccuracies in the measurement.

D. The cardiac output is assessed by measuring the area under the temperature change curve.

E. Cardiac output measurements will be unchanged by wedging of the pulmonary artery catheter.

QUESTION 42

Charcoal is effective in the following drug overdoses

A. Malathion pesticide.

B. Iron.

C. Diazepam.

D. Theophylline.

E. Cyanide.

QUESTION 43

Verapamil

A. Is a derivative of papaverine.
B. Is almost completely absorbed after oral administration.
C. Has a bioavailability following oral administration of about 75%.
D. Is highly bound to plasma proteins.
E. Is largely excreted by the gastro-intestinal tract.

QUESTION 44

Rocuronium

A. Is more potent than vecuronium.
B. Is chemically related to vecuronium.
C. In suitable doses produces good intubating conditions in 60–90 s.
D. Has a longer elimination half time than vecuronium.
E. Possesses active metabolites.

QUESTION 45

Cerebral blood flow

A. Is dependent on intracranial pressure.
B. Is decreased by hypoxia.
C. Is increased by standing up from lying.
D. Is approximately 750 ml/min in a 70 kg man.
E. Can be measured using the Fick principle.

QUESTION 46

Gastric emptying

A. Is slow after a fat rich meal.
B. Is increased due to the entero-gastric reflex.
C. Is passive following vagotomy.
D. Is reduced by cholecystokinin.
E. Is controlled by the pylorus.

QUESTION 47

The arterio-venous O_2 difference

A. Is increased in sepsis.
B. Is increased when the balloon of a pulmonary artery catheter is inflated.
C. Is decreased in cyanide toxicity.
D. Is increased in low cardiac output states.
E. Is normally 10 ml O_2 / dl.

QUESTION 48

5-Hydroxytryptamine (5-HT)

A. Is synthesised principally from dietary tryptamine.
B. Is located in intestine, neutrophils and the CNS.
C. Is synthesised from a precursor derived from dietary sources.
D. Undergoes deamination by enzymes located exclusively in the liver.
E. Is metabolised principally to 5 hydroxyindoleacetic acid (5-HIAA).

QUESTION 49

Hyperkalaemia following suxamethonium administration

A. Is abolished by precurarisation.
B. Is normally of the order of 0.5-1 mmol/l.
C. Is more marked in patients suffering from acute oliguric renal failure.
D. Is more marked in patients with chronic renal failure.
E. May be severe for as long as six months following a large burn.

QUESTION 50

An oxygen cylinder

A. Should have a filling ratio of 0.67.
B. Is painted black with a black and white shoulder in the UK.
C. Should never be turned on unless connected to the anaesthetic machine.
D. Has a plastic collar to identify the date of filling.
E. Has a valve that must be greased before attaching it to the anaesthetic machine.

QUESTION 51

The standard deviation of a normally distributed population

A. Is the square root of the variance.
B. Is small in a distribution curve with a tall peak.
C. Defines limits above and below the mean containing about two thirds of the population.
D. Is greater than the standard error of the mean.
E. Defines the range of the population.

QUESTION 52

Iron within the human body

A. Is bound predominantly as haemoglobin.
B. Is transported principally as ferritin.
C. Is excreted renally.
D. Is shed into the intestinal lumen.
E. Is absorbed mainly in the ferrous form.

QUESTION 53

Concerning the pharmacokinetics of theophylline

A. It has a long plasma half life.

B. It accumulates in patients with renal impairment.

C. Interactions occur with drugs metabolised by the cytochrome P_{450} enzyme system.

D. The rate of metabolism is substantially increased in smokers.

E. Concomitant administration of phenobarbitone may alter dose requirements.

QUESTION 54

Epidural analgesia in obstetrics is absolutely contraindicated in the following condition

A. Aortic stenosis.

B. Left ventricular failure.

C. Pulmonary hypertension.

D. Placenta praevia.

E. Previous spinal surgery.

QUESTION 55

With regard to ketamine

A. It is metabolised to the inactive metabolite norketamine.

B. Less than 5% is excreted in the urine unchanged.

C. It is painful on intravenous injection.

D. It is a potent cerebral vasodilator.

E. It lowers the seizure threshold in epileptic patients.

QUESTION 56

Comparing lignocaine with prilocaine

A. Lignocaine has a higher pKa.

B. Lignocaine is more extensively protein bound.

C. Lignocaine is more potent.

D. Lignocaine has a lower molecular weight.

E. Lignocaine is less lipid soluble.

QUESTION 57

Bioavailability of an orally administered drug depends on

A. Water solubility.

B. Lipid solubility.

C. The presence of other drugs in the lumen of the gut.

D. First pass metabolism.

E. Dose of drug.

QUESTION 58

Fibrinolysis

A. Is usually increased after surgery.
B. May be increased by venous occlusion.
C. May occur in association with malignancy.
D. Rarely follows disseminated intravascular coagulopathy.
E. Activation involves clotting factors IX and X.

QUESTION 59

Impedance

A. Is made up of reactance and resistance.
B. May be used to measure gastric emptying.
C. Is the resistance of a coil to changing voltage.
D. Is used to measure rapid changes in cardiac output.
E. Is useful for calibrating other blood flow measurements.

QUESTION 60

The sulphonylurea class of drugs

A. Are effective in type I diabetes.
B. May cause an upgrading of insulin receptors.
C. Have lactic acidosis as a recognised complication.
D. Includes drugs that bind extensively to plasma proteins.
E. May need to be replaced by insulin as tolerance develops after prolonged use.

QUESTION 61

Postoperative shivering

A. Is due to the use of volatile anaesthetic agents.
B. May cause hypoxia in recovery.
C. May be arrested by a single dose of 25 mg pethidine intravenously.
D. Does not occur after spinal anaesthesia.
E. The incidence of shivering with extradural analgesia is reduced by the concurrent use of an opiate.

QUESTION 62

The following are SI units

A. Litre (l)
B. Millimetres of mercury (mmHg).
C. Ohm
D. Candela (Cd).
E. Bar (bar)

QUESTION 63

Interruption of the cervical sympathetic chain causes

A. Enophthalmos.
B. Mydriasis.
C. Complete ptosis.
D. Ipsilateral hyperhydrosis.
E. Nasal mucosal engorgement.

QUESTION 64

Concerning the properties of cardiac tissue

A. Myocardial cells have a RMP of -70 mV.
B. Myocardial cells possess gap junctions.
C. The RMP of pacemaker cells is slightly lower than that of atrial muscle.
D. The bundle-branch conducting tissue has the longest plateau phase.
E. The AV node is mainly supplied by the left Xth nerve.

QUESTION 65

In the EEG, delta waves occur

A. Upon closing the eyes.
B. Normally in children.
C. Prominently over the frontal area.
D. With increased cortical activity.
E. Normally during sleep.

QUESTION 66

The following are correct definitions

A. 1 mol Ca^{2+} = 2 eq Ca^{2+}.
B. Osmolality = the concentration of osmotically active particles in a solution.
C. Anatomical dead space can never be greater than physiological dead space.
D. The mass of substance freely filtered by a glomerulus is the product of the GFR, time, and the plasma concentration of that substance.
E. Free water clearance is the difference between the urine volume and the clearance of osmoles.

QUESTION 67

The following are recognised complications of the long term administration of amiodarone

A. Prologation of the Q-T interval.
B. Peripheral neuropathy.
C. Disorders of thyroid function.
D. Reversible restrictive lung defect.
E. Optic atrophy.

QUESTION 68

Soda lime

A. Absorbs 250 litres of carbon dioxide per kilogram of fresh soda lime.
B. Phenolphthalein indicator is pink when fresh and white when exhausted.
C. Is normally sized 4-8 mesh.
D. Soda lime dust is inert but may cause a sarcoid-like disease in the lungs.
E. A warm canister indicates that the soda lime is still working.

QUESTION 69

During pregnancy

A. HCG levels reach a maximum during the first trimester.
B. Progesterone levels are maximal during the third trimester.
C. Secretion of progesterone ceases on the first day postpartum.
D. Progesterone inhibits aldosterone activity
E. Oestradiol reduces the plasma cholesterol.

QUESTION 70

Heat loss

A. Conduction is the largest factor in patient heat loss.
B. Radiation accounts for about 10% of the total heat loss.
C. Convection is due to heating of the adjacent air layer which is replaced by cooler air from the surroundings.
D. Heat lost in breathing dry gases is approximately 15% of total heat loss in the anaesthetised subject.
E. Burns from faulty heating equipment are more likely in the vasoconstricted patient.

QUESTION 71

Concerning osmolality

A. Plasma osmolality is approximately 285 milliosmoles per litre.
B. Renal medullary osmolality is reduced by increased vasa recta blood flow.
C. Hypothalamic receptors play a part in its regulation.
D. A rise in serum osmolality results in release of ADH from the anterior pituitary.
E. Salt deficit is accompanied by rises in plasma levels of renin, angiotensin II, aldosterone and ADH.

QUESTION 72

The National Confidential Enquiry into Perioperative Deaths (NCEPOD)

A. Considers death in hospital within 28 days of surgery.
B. Represents a research project exploring death in hospital.
C. Considers in detail every death in hospital within the stipulated time.
D. In addition to presenting data makes recommendations on running surgical services.
E. There is a legal requirement to complete the NCEPOD form if one is sent to you.

QUESTION 73

These are appropriate statistical methods

A. The Mann-Whitney test for comparison of quantity of surgical blood loss with or without use of a tourniquet.
B. The Chi-squared test in the comparison of whether patients left the intensive care unit alive or dead.
C. ANOVA for comparison of multiple groups and reduction of blood pressure.
D. Student's t-test for difference in height between groups of infants.
E. Student's t-test for evaluating difference between baldness among Conservative and Labour politicians.

QUESTION 74

Non-invasive measurement of blood pressure

A. Was first described using an occluding cuff in 1796.
B. The diastolic pressure is recorded as the pressure at which the first muffling of the sound occurs.
C. When using a mercury sphygmomanometer the space above the column will be a virtual vacuum.
D. Requires a cuff that is wider than the diameter of the arm.
E. Tends to give a lower diastolic pressure than direct means.

QUESTION 75

When using a train of four to monitor a non-depolarising block

A. The stimulator should deliver four supramaximal stimuli at 4 Hz.
B. The fourth twitch (T4) will be smaller than the first twitch (T1).
C. Post-tetanic fascilitation is due to accumulation of acetylcholine (ACh) in the synaptic cleft.
D. The response to muscle relaxants of the facial muscles is similar to that of the diaphragm.
E. Presence of all four twitches indicates a patient who is adequately reversed for extubation.

QUESTION 76

Concerning central venous cannulation

A. The Seldinger technique depends on passage of the cannula over the needle.
B. The internal jugular vein is accessible by a needle inserted at the level of C6 aiming towards the contralateral nipple.
C. The right sided approach avoids the risk of traumatising the thoracic duct.
D. Pneumothorax is a hazard of the subclavian approach.
E. The femoral vein lies lateral to the artery.

QUESTION 77

The following are examples of monosynaptic reflexes

A. The withdrawal reflex.
B. The "knee jerk" patellar reflex.
C. The inverse stretch reflex.
D. The cremasteric reflex.
E. The corneal reflex.

QUESTION 78

Anaesthesia breathing circuits

A. The Lack circuit is a Mapleson D system.
B. The Magill attachment is more efficient for spontaneous breathing than for controlled ventilation.
C. The recommended fresh gas flow rate for controlled ventilation through a Bain circuit is 70 ml/kg body weight.
D. Minimum fresh gas flow to avoid rebreathing using a Mapleson A is equal to that patient's minute ventilation.
E. The Mapleson F system is a modification of the Mapleson E system.

QUESTION 79

During salicylate poisoning

A. Free salicylate is excreted in a pH dependant fashion from the kidney.

B. The normal de-sulphation process becomes saturated.

C. There is commonly a respiratory alkalosis.

D. There may be hypoglycaemia.

E. Hyperkalaemia is common.

QUESTION 80

Concerning midazolam

A. The parenteral preparation is buffered to an acidic pH.

B. The parenteral preparation is formulated in propylene glycol.

C. It is highly lipid soluble at physiological pH.

D. About 50% is excreted unchanged in the urine.

E. It undergoes conjugation to produce compounds which have pharmacological activity.

QUESTION 81

With regard to mivacurium

A. It is formulated as an aqueous solution of the chloride salt.

B. The solution is basic.

C. The shelf-life of the solution is approximately 6 months.

D. It is a short-acting benzyl–isoquinolinium depolarising neuromuscular blocking agent.

E. It is broken down by esterification by plasma cholinesterase.

QUESTION 82

Concerning the knee jerk reflex

A. It is monosynaptic.

B. The synaptic transmitter is aspartate.

C. The sensory organ is the muscle spindle.

D. It involves spinal roots L2,3,4.

E. Glycine inhibition occurs in fibres to antagonistic muscles.

QUESTION 83

Regarding the Harvard minimum monitoring standards

A. These were instituted by a group of clinicians to reduce malpractice premiums.

B. They allow for the patient to be left with a suitably qualified trained technical assistant.

C. Vital signs must be recorded every 10 minutes.

D. They call for monitoring of ventilation which may be by direct observation of the reservoir bag.

E. They specifically require the use of pulse oximetry.

QUESTION 84

Concerning the cranial nerves

A. VII provides taste sensation to the posterior third of the tongue.

B. V provides motor fibres to the jaw and tongue.

C. V provides sensation to the cornea.

D. VII provides sensation to the forehead.

E. VII is required for the corneal reflex.

QUESTION 85

Concerning the enteric nervous system

A. It contains pre-ganglionic cholinergic fibres.

B. Vagal fibres are post-ganglionic.

C. It contains post-ganglionic sympathetic fibres.

D. Many sympathetic fibres end on cholinergic neurones.

E. Many sympathetic fibres end directly on intestinal smooth muscle.

QUESTION 86

Breathing spontaneously in the lateral position

A. Perfusion is greater in the dependent lung.

B. Ventilation is decreased in the uppermost lung.

C. V/Q is higher in the dependent lung.

D. Dependent lung has a lower PO_2.

E. Non-dependent lung has a higher PCO_2.

QUESTION 87

Liver blood flow

A. Is normally 25% of cardiac output.

B. Via the portal system accounts for 30% of the total blood supply to the liver.

C. From the hepatic and portal systems drains via the lobular veins into the hepatic veins.

D. Is controlled by noradrenergic mediated vasoconstriction of the portal vessels.

E. In the portal vein is normally at a pressure of 10 mmHg.

QUESTION 88

The American Society of Anesthesiologists (ASA) Physical Status

A. Predicts postoperative outcome.

B. Was instituted in response to malpractice claims.

C. ASA Class II would include a well-controlled asthmatic.

D. ASA Class IV indicates a condition which impedes activity but does not represent a threat to life.

E. Postscript E indicates an elective case.

QUESTION 89

Dantrolene

A. Can be given orally for the prophylaxis of malignant hyperthermia (MH)
B. When given intravenously for the treatment of MH, the initial dose is 10 mg/kg
C. Can precipitate respiratory failure
D. Affects neuromuscular transmission
E. Is formulated in combination with mannitol

QUESTION 90

Renal clearance of a drug

A. Is dependent upon urine flow rate.
B. Will be about 750 ml/min for a drug that is passively filtered and not reabsorbed.
C. Equals renal plasma flow if the drug is completely secreted into the proximal tubule and not reabsorbed.
D. Equals mass of drug excreted divided by time.
E. Equals urine output for a highly lipophilic drug.

Exam 1: Answers

ANSWER 1

A. FALSE   B. FALSE   C.TRUE   D. FALSE   E. TRUE

Normal values are COHb 0.2-2% (although it may be up to 6% in smokers); MetHb < 1%; OxyHb 70% (in peripheral venous blood); free Hb 0.00001-0.00004%; HbA2 2%.

Ref: Yentis, Hirsch, Smith. Anaesthesia A to Z. Butterworth-Heinemann

ANSWER 2

A. TRUE   B. TRUE   C. FALSE   D. TRUE   E. FALSE

The order of efficiency of the nebulisers with normal values is (from the least to the greatest):

Gas bubbled through cold water.

HME Normal upper trachea (33 g/m^3).

Heated water bath 100% saturation at 37° (44 g/m^3).

Heated nebulizer with anvil.

Ultrasonic nebulizer (approx. 200% saturation at 37°C).

Ref: Davis PD, Parbrook GD, Kenny GNC. Basic Physics and Measurement in Anaesthesia, 4th edn. Butterworth-Heinemann, 1995

ANSWER 3

A. FALSE   B. TRUE   C. FALSE   D.TRUE   E. TRUE

There are currently three types of opioid receptors described. Sigma receptor effects are not reversed by naloxone, and it cannot therefore be classified as an opioid receptor. Activation causes a decrease in neurotransmission. Endogenous ligands include enkephalin, dynorphin, and probably beta-endorphin. Suprisingly, the presence of opioid receptors has been described in the knee joint.

Ref: British Journal of Anaesthesia 1994; 73: 132-134

ANSWER 4

A. FALSE   B. FALSE   C. TRUE   D.TRUE   E. FALSE

ANSWER 5

A. TRUE   B. TRUE   C. TRUE   D.TRUE   E. FALSE

CO=HR x SV. Stroke volume is increased by increased contractility (dp/dt), and increased

ventricular filling (increasing LVEDV, eg by increasing pulmonary venous pressure.)
Increasing aortic pressure will decrease SV.

Ref: Ganong WF. Review of Medical Physiology. Lange.

ANSWER 6

A. TRUE   B. FALSE   C. TRUE   D. TRUE   E. TRUE

Electrical defibrillation is the treatment of choice for ventricular fibrillation. Outcome
from defibrillation is most significantly affected by the time from onset of VF to first
defibrillation. Other factors affecting outcome include acidosis, hypoxia, hypothermia,
drug toxicity (e.g. digoxin) or electrolyte imbalance. Other rhythms (asystole and idioven-
tricular rhythms) are more resistant to defibrillation than VF. As air is a poor conductor of
electricity the smaller cushion of air between the paddles and the heart in end-expiration
produces a more successful outcome.

Ref: Faust RJ (ed) Anesthesiology Review, 2nd edn. Churchill Livingstone, 1994

ANSWER 7

A. FALSE   B. TRUE   C. FALSE   D. TRUE   E. TRUE

Magnesium is the fourth most plentiful cation (approximately 1000 mmol in a 70 kg man).
50-60% is in bone. Magnesium balance is achieved by absorption through the gut and renal
excretion.

Ref: Ganong WF. Review of Medical Physiology. Lange

ANSWER 8

A. FALSE   B. TRUE   C. TRUE   D. TRUE   E. TRUE

Confidence intervals describe the range of values around a mean, an odds ratio, a p
value or a standard deviation within which the true value lies. A confidence interval which
is narrow emphasises the significance of the result, but it is the p value which describes
significance, not the confidence intervals around it.

ANSWER 9

A. TRUE   B. TRUE   C. FALSE   D. TRUE   E. FALSE

Renal blood flow is normally 25% cardiac output and is maintained by autoregulation
whilst mean arterial pressure remains in the range 80-200 mmHg (even in the denervated
kidney). Macula densa cells are found in the distal tubule. Renal oxygen consumption is
only approximately 18 ml/min.

Ref: Despopoulos A, Silbernagl S. Color Atlas of Physiology. 120-150

ANSWER 10

A. TRUE   B. TRUE   C. TRUE   D. TRUE   E. FALSE

Insulin is a 51 amino acid peptide formed by removal of the C-chain from proinsulin.
The insulin receptor is composed of two alpha subunits and two transmembranal beta
subunits. Insulin binding leads to internalisation of the hormone:receptor complex.

Ref: Despopoulos A, Silbernagl S. Color Atlas of Physiology. 110-118

ANSWER   11

A. TRUE   B. TRUE   C. FALSE   D. TRUE   E. FALSE

The placenta can produce steroid hormones but requires a blood borne supply of cholesterol as a substrate. The male hormones (androgens) are all 19 C molecules (female sex hormones = 18 C, gluco & mineralocorticoids = 21 C). The adrenal cortex contains 17-, 21-, and 11-hydroxylases. Hydroxylation at C atom 21 first renders the steroid molecule immune to later 17-hydroxylase attack and these all become mineralocorticoids. However, if 17-hydroxylation occurs first, synthesis can continue either to glucocorticoids which may still be 21-hydroxylated or the 17-ketosteroids.

Ref: Despopoulos A, Silbernagl S. Color Atlas of Physiology, 232-271

ANSWER   12

A. TRUE   B. TRUE   C. FALSE   D. TRUE   E. FALSE

Non-parametric tests are used for data that is not normally distributed and data where the distribution is unknown. It can be applied to normally distributed data as well. Student's paired t-test is a parametric test applied to two groups and is more powerful than the standard t-test if the same subjects are examined before and after treatment.

Ref: Yentis, Hirsch, Smith. Anaesthesia A to Z. Butterworth-Heinemann

ANSWER   13

A. FALSE   B. TRUE   C. FALSE   D. TRUE   E. TRUE

The proton pump involves ATP-driven Na:K exchange and passive HCO_3(out) for Cl(in) exchange at the capillary:cell membrane. Passive K^+ and Cl^- loss into the gastric lumen is accompanied by ATP-driven K^+ reabsorption in exchange for excreted H^+ ions. Gastrin comes from G-cells.

Ref: Despopoulos A, Silbernagl S. Color Atlas of Physiology. 208

ANSWER   14

A. TRUE   B. FALSE   C. TRUE   D. TRUE   E. FALSE

Succinyl monocholine is weakly active. Codeine is metabolised to morphine. Propranolol is metabolised to 4-hydroxy propranolol; phenobarbitone is the active metabolite of primidone.

ANSWER   15

A. TRUE   B. FALSE   C. FALSE   D. FALSE   E. FALSE

Smokers are more likely to desaturate in recovery, as are the passive-smoking children of smoking parents. Carboxyhaemoglobin is distinguished from oxyhaemoglobin by bench co-oximetry and not pulse oximetry. A heavy smoker with a carboxyhaemoglobin level of 15% cannot have a maximal oxyhaemoglobin saturation of 85% on room air, since the other effects of smoking include V/Q mismatch, sputum retention and other causes of hypoxaemia. He or she might manage 85% on 100% oxygen. Carboxyhaemaglobin absorbs as much light as oxyhaemaglobin and so overestimates the true arterial saturation when measured with pulse oximetry. Twelve hours' abstinence restores oxygen carriage to that of the non-smoker but airway hypersensitivity persists for 8 weeks or more.

ANSWER 16

A. FALSE   B. FALSE   C. TRUE   D. TRUE   E. FALSE

Reduction in blood volume causes reduced baroreceptor stretch, therefore increased sympathetic output. This causes generalised vasoconstriction but spares the vessels of the brain and the heart. In the kidneys the efferent arterioles constrict more than the afferent. Stagnant hypoxia causes increased chemoreceptor discharge.

Ref: Ganong WF. Review of Medical Physiology. Lange. Ch33

ANSWER 17

A. TRUE   B. TRUE   C. FALSE   D. TRUE   E. FALSE

Bacteriostasis is the inhibition of bacterial replication as opposed to bactericidal activity which kills the organisms.

Bactericidal groups include:

Penicillins

Cephalosporins and other beta lactams

Aminoglycocides

Vancomycin

Bacteriostatic groups include:

Macrolides

Tetracyclines

Sulphonamides/trimethoprim (bactericidal if used in combination) Metronidazole

Chloramphenicol

ANSWER 18

A. FALSE   B. TRUE   C. TRUE   D. FALSE   E. TRUE

The HME is a cheap, convenient humidifier that contains a metal or paper mesh on which the exhaled humidity can condense and evaporate. The HME can be made hygroscopic (moisture-retaining) and impregnated with a bactericide. Some HMEs are effective as viral filters. The performance of the filter is reduced by increased tidal volumes as there is less time for the condensation-evaporation cycle to occur. Performance also starts to deteriorate after the first few hours.

Ref: Dorsch JA, Dorsch SE. Understanding Anesthesia Equipment; Construction, Care and Complications, 2nd edn. Williams & Wilkins, 1984

ANSWER 19

A. TRUE   B. FALSE   C. FALSE   D. TRUE   E. FALSE

Respiratory patients should not be sedated and adjunctive analgesic techniques which avoid or reduce the opiate requirement are valuable. Postoperative myocardial infarction associated with hypoxia is commonest on the second and third nights. Breathlessness at rest and resting PaO_2 <7.2 kPa are the best predictors of the need for postoperative ventilation, but apparently alarming pulmonary function tests have been shown to be compatible with safe general anaesthesia. Cor pulmonale is the onset of right ventricular failure due to pulmonary hypertension as a result of lung disease.

Ref: Nunn. Anaesthesia 1988;43;543

ANSWER 20

A. FALSE   B. FALSE   C. FALSE   D. TRUE   E. FALSE

Diamorphine is a synthetic morphine derivative which does not itself bind to opioid receptors, but is rapidly hydrolysed to the active metabolites 6-monoacetylmorphine and morphine. It is highly lipid soluble. It is extensively absorbed when administered orally. Bioavailability is low due to first pass metabolism.

PHYSICAL: 40% protein bound, Vd 350 litres

Ref: Sasada, Smith. Drugs in Anaesthesia and Intensive Care

ANSWER 21

A. FALSE   B. FALSE   C. FALSE   D. FALSE   E. TRUE

The rate of drug transfer may be described by the equation:$dC/dT = - k.C^n$.

dC/dT = the rate at which the concentration gradient declines

k = a constant

n = the exponent of C with value 1 or 0

A first order process means a constant PROPORTION of drug is transfered in unit time.

A zero order process implies a constant AMOUNT of drug is transfered in unit time.

First order processes occur when $dC/dT = -k.C$. At any time, the rate is directly proportional to the concentration. The first order rate constant is the proportion by which C declines in time T at the actual value of C. Zero order kinetics, on the other hand, apply when an active process is saturated such that $dC/dT = k$. The rate of transfer is independent of C because n=0.

Ref: Nimmo, Rowbotham, Smith. Anaesthesia, Blackwell, chapter 15

ANSWER 22

A. FALSE   B. TRUE   C. FALSE   D. FALSE   E. TRUE

Nitric oxide is also produced by macrophages and thrombocytes. There are two types of NO synthase, a calcium dependent and a calcium independent form. It is synthesised from L-arginine. The haemoglobin molecule has an affinity 1500 times higher to NO than to CO. Nitrosyl haemoglobin is produced, which in the presence of oxygen, is oxidised to methaemoglobin. Nitrate is ultimately produced after regeneration of haemoglobin by methaemoglobin reductase in red blood cells.

Inhaled NO improves oxygenation in patients with ARDS by pulmonary vasodilatation in areas of ventilated alveoli, thus diverting blood flow away from areas of intrapulmonary shunt to areas of more normal V/Q ratio. NO is rapidly de-activated in blood and systemic hypotension does not occur. Conversely, following the use of systemically applied vasodilators such as prostacyclin and sodium nitroprusside, there may be an increase in shunt and a fall in systemic pressure and oxygen tension.

Ref: British Journal of Anaesthesia 1995; 74: 443

ANSWER 23

A. TRUE   B. TRUE   C. FALSE   D. TRUE   E. TRUE

The ventricular muscle action potential is formed by an increase in Na^+ permeability, followed by Ca^{++} permeability, followed by K^+ permeability. The characteristic plateau phase is caused by calcium permeability. There is no prepotential decay (only pacemaker cells have this). The prolonged refractory period prevents tetany. Resting membrane potential (normally -80 mV) is dependent on extracellular K^+ concentration. Action potential magnitude is Na^+ dependent

Ref: Ganong WF. Review of Medical Physiology. Lange, Ch3

ANSWER   24
A. FALSE   B. TRUE   C. FALSE   D. TRUE   E. TRUE

Excitation is normally initiated from the SA node and spreads through both atria to the AV node. Via two branches of the bundle of His it reaches the purkinje network which conveys the impulse to ventricular muscle. Activation then takes place from endo- to epicardium and from the apex to the base.

Chronotropism = the frequency with which impulses are initiated in the pacemaker.

Dromotropism = the speed of conduction of excitation.

Ref: Despopoulos A, Silbernagl S. Color Atlas of Physiology, 154-190

ANSWER   25
A. FALSE   B. TRUE   C. TRUE   D. TRUE   E. FALSE

REM sleep cycles lasting 10-40 minutes occur every 90 minutes. During REM sleep alpha wave activity (8-13 Hz) is seen on the EEG. A 3 Hz spike + wave pattern is typical of petit mal epilepsy. ACTH and cortisol levels fall consistently throughout the day reaching a minimum at about midnight. Thereafter, they rise until about 6am.

Ref: Despopoulos A, Silbernagl S. Color Atlas of Physiology, 260 & 292

ANSWER   26
A. TRUE   B. TRUE   C. FALSE   D. TRUE   E. FALSE

Tachyphylaxis is tolerance that develops rapidly.

ANSWER   27
A. TRUE   B. FALSE   C. FALSE   D. FALSE   E. TRUE

MAC is reduced by about 7% per degree centigrade of temperature reduction. Sex, duration of anaesthesia and alcoholism have no effect. Hypothyroidism is associated with an increased sensitivity to anaesthetic agents. The MAC of a volatile agent is reduced in the presence of other anaesthetic and analgesic agents as is expected. For convenience MAC is described as volume percent but refers to the partial pressure of the agent in the brain. This is important when considering the effect of changes in altitude in vaporiser function.

ANSWER   28
A. FALSE   B. TRUE   C. TRUE   D. TRUE   E. FALSE

FENTANYL
Equipotent dose = 0.1 mg
% ionized at pH 7.4 = 91%
% protein bound = 80%
Clearance = 0.8-1.3 litres/min

Vd =20-400 litres

ALFENTANIL

Equipotent dose = 0.5 mg

% ionized at pH 7.4 = 11%

% protein bound = 90%

Clearance = 0.2-0.6 litres/min

Vd =9-40 litres

Ref: Nimmo & Smith. Anaesthesia. Blackwell

ANSWER   29

A. FALSE   B. FALSE   C. FALSE   D. FALSE   E. FALSE

Naturally occuring fatty acids have an even number of Cs. FFAs are bound to albumin; cholesterol, triglycerides, and phospholipids are transported as lipoprotein complexes. Lipoprotein lipase breaks triglycerides into FFA & glycerol. VLDLs are broken down into IDLs and LDLs (main cholesterol carrier). Beta-oxidation involves repeated 2C-chain cleavage.

Ref: Ganong WF. Review of Medical Physiology. Lange, Ch17

ANSWER   30

A. FALSE   B. FALSE   C. FALSE   D. FALSE   E. TRUE

Disinfection (not decontamination) implies the removal or killing of most or all infective organisms, but not spores. It is the level of cleaning commonly used for anaesthetic equipment that does not come into direct contact with the patient. It may be performed by heat or chemical means. The latter include alcohol solutions though these should not be used for electrically-powered ventilators because of the risk of explosions. Hypochlorite is useful as it is highly effective against a number of viruses including HIV. Sterilisation in theatres is normally by autoclaving, though gluteraldehyde can be usd for both disinfection and sterilisation. Gamma irradiation requires a large, expensive unit and is used for commercial sterilisation of disposable items.

Ref: Davey A, Moyle JTB, Ward CS. Ward's Anaesthetic Equipment, 3rd edn. W.B. Saunders, 1992

ANSWER   31

A. FALSE   B. TRUE   C. FALSE   D. FALSE   E. FALSE

Diabetics are unsuitable for day surgery, as are patients with malignant hyperpyrexia; suxamathonium apnoeas are not. While gastro-oesophageal reflux is not a contraindication per se, the usual precautions regarding airway safety need to be applied and if the patient with reflux is extremely obese, then he or she would be excluded for that reason. Regionals are not contraindicated but the patient needs to walk safely and have passed urine before discharge; many anaesthetists use caudal analgesia for day case circumcision, for example. Using a cooker is specifically prohibited in the first 24 hours, as is child minding in addition to driving and operating machinery.

ANSWER   32

A. FALSE   B. TRUE   C. FALSE   D. FALSE   E. FALSE

It is useful by the intravenous route only, when rapid short-lived beta-blockade is required.

It is rapidly metabolised by red-cell esterases and is non-selective.

Ref: Drugs and Therapeutics Bulletin 1996; 34 (7) July

ANSWER 33

A. TRUE   B. TRUE   C. TRUE   D. TRUE   E. TRUE

Gas flowing through a constriction will produce a negative pressure as it expands after the constriction. This allows entrainment of gas or liquid in a predictable manner. This is the Venturi principle and is fundamental to much anaesthetic equipment. The 'Ventimask' allows delivery of a constant oxygen percentage at variable inspiratory flow rates. The production of a low pressure by an injector can be used for suction or scavenging devices. Nebulisers may be used for drug delivery and for humidification, and the jet ventilator (such as the Carden device or Sanders injector) relies on air entrainment to assist ventilation.

Ref: Davey A., Moyle JTB, Ward CS. Ward's Anaesthetic Equipment, 3rd edn. W.B. Saunders, 1992

ANSWER 34

A. FALSE   B. FALSE   C. TRUE   D. TRUE   E. TRUE

Methohexitone is a methylated oxybarbituate. It is a white powder made up into a 1% solution. The pH of the solution is 11 and the pKa is 7.9. It is more potent than thiopentone and usually admininistered intravenously at a dose of 1-1.5 mg/kg. It is 75% non ionised at pH 7.4 and onset of action is faster than for thiopentone. Recovery is in 2-3 minutes and it has a shorter duration of action than thiopentone due to a very short distribution half life and high clearance (4x thiopentone). It may cause paradoxical excitation at low dose. It has no active metabolites unlike thiopentone.

Ref: Sasada, Smith. Drugs in Anaesthesia and Intensive Care

ANSWER 35

A. FALSE   B. FALSE   C. TRUE   D. TRUE   E. TRUE

The increase in intrathoracic pressure imposed by the inspiratory phase of IPPV, added to a degree of cardiac tamponade and increased pulmonary vascular resistance, conspire to reduce venous return and so decrease cardiac output. This reduction in cardiac output added to activation of the renin-angiotensin-aldosterone system causes a decrease in urine generation, not a diuresis, although this is seen on withdrawal of ventilatory support. Cerebral perfusion pressure falls because of increased venous pressure and reduced mean arterial pressure; neurosurgical patients are ventilated to reduce arterial CO_2 and paralysed to reduce straining and so reduce intracranial pressure. Inotropic support is frequently employed in these patients to overcome the effects of IPPV and to preserve mean arterial pressure even in the presence of a normally functioning cardiovascular system. Dead space increases because of the tracheal tube and connections.

Ref: Nunn, Utting, Burnell Brown. General Anaesthesia, Butterworth-Heinemann

ANSWER 36

A. TRUE   B. FALSE   C. TRUE   D. TRUE   E. FALSE

The Quetelet index (or body mass index) is weight (kg) divided by the square of height (in m^2). The upper limit of normal is 24.9. Overweight is 25-29.9, obese is 30-34.9, and morbid obesity over 35. Hypertension, ischaemic heart disease and increased oxygen consumption are characteristics, as are airway obstruction, right heart strain and, eventually, pulmonary hypertension and right-sided failure. The FRC is reduced with a tendency to V/Q mismatch and hypoxaemia. Hiatus hernia with reflux, and diabetes are other considerations.

Ref: Shenkman et al. Perioperative management of the obese patient. British Journal of Anaesthesia 1993;70:349.

ANSWER 37
A. TRUE   B. FALSE   C. TRUE   D. FALSE   E. FALSE

During pregnancy minute volume increases by 50% in the first trimester, (thought to be a central effect due to increased progesterone) and mainly caused by increased tidal volume. Maternal $PaCO_2$ decreases to ~ 4 KPa but renal bicarbonate retention keeps pH normal. FRC is reduced by upward displacement of the diaphragm by the gravid uterus (both ERV and RV are decreased.)

Ref: Yentis, Hirsch, Smith. Anaesthesia A to Z. Butterworth-Heinemann

ANSWER 38
A. TRUE   B. FALSE   C. FALSE   D. TRUE   E. TRUE

Latent heat of vaporisation is the energy required to change a liquid to vapour at a constant temperature. It is defined at specified temperature as it decreases as the temperature increases. When the temperature reaches the critical temperature the energy required to vaporise the liquid is zero (vaporisation occurs spontaneously) and above this the substance cannot exist as a liquid. Ethyl chloride has been used as a topical anaesthetic. Its action relies on the cooling effect of the vaporising liquid impeding conduction in sensory nerves. Vaporisation of volatile anaesthetic agents requires energy to overcome the latent heat. This is provided by the cooling of the body of the vaporiser and the agent within. As the liquid cools its saturated vapour pressure (svp) falls so the concentration leaving the vaporisation chamber is smaller. This requires compensation to increase the proportion of the fresh gas flow passing through the chamber as the temperature falls.

Ref: Davis PD, Parbrook GD, Kenny GNC. Basic Physics and Measurement in Anaesthesia, 4th edn. Butterworth-Heinemann, 1995

ANSWER 39
A. TRUE   B. TRUE   C. FALSE   D. TRUE   E. TRUE

Bronchial muscle: PGF2alpha contracts, PGE2 relaxes. GI secretion: PGE2 inhibits. Uterus: PGE2 and PGF2alpha contract. Kidney: PGE2 and PGI2 provoke natriuresis. CNS: fever. Pain: PGE2 and PGI2 sensitize nociceptive nerve endings. Platelets: TXA2 causes aggregation, PGI2 inhibits.

Ref: Despopoulos A, Silbernagl S. Color Atlas of Physiology, 232-271

ANSWER 40
A. FALSE   B. FALSE   C. TRUE   D. FALSE   E. TRUE

It is a coumarin derivative. It inhibits the synthesis of factors II, VII, IX & X. It is bound to albumin and not the globulin fraction.

ANSWER 41

A. TRUE   **B. FALSE**   **C. TRUE**   **D. TRUE**   **E. FALSE**

The thermodilution technique using a pulmonary artery catheter gives an accurate, repeatable measurement of cardiac output. The cardiac output is assessed by measuring the area under the curve temperature change recorded at the distal end of the catheter by a thermistor. Injection should be performed smoothly over less than 4 seconds. Inaccuracies may occur due to:

Patient factors (including right heart valvular abnormalities, intracardiac shunts, arrhythmias and respiration).

Injectate factors (too little injectate will lead to an over-estimation, errors in injectate temperature measurement or prolonged injection duration).

Thermistor factors (wedging or partial wedging of the catheter produces unreliable results as the cooled mixture does not make adequate contact with the thermistor; looping of the catheter reduces the distance between the injection port and the thermistor so mixing of the injectate with blood may be incomplete; thrombi on the catheter will produce under-estimates of cardiac output).

Ref: Faust RJ (ed) Anesthesiology Review, 2nd edn. Churchill Livingstone, 1994

ANSWER 42

A. FALSE   **B. FALSE**   **C. TRUE**   **D. TRUE**   **E. FALSE**

Drugs that are well adsorbed by activated charcoal include the following:
Barbituates
Anticonvulsants
Antidepressants
Benzodiazepines
Theophylline.

Ref: Management of acute poisioning. British Journal of Anaesthesia 1993; 70: 562

ANSWER 43

A. TRUE   **B. .TRUE**   **C. FALSE**   **D. TRUE**   **E. FALSE**

Verapamil is a synthetic papaverine derivative. Although well absorbed following oral administration, it undergoes extensive first pass metabolism in the liver, and therefore bioavailability is only about 10-20%. 70% of metabolites are excreted by the kidney.

Ref: Sasada, Smith. Drugs in Anaesthesia & Intensive Care

ANSWER 44

A. FALSE   **B. TRUE**   **C. TRUE**   **D. TRUE**   **E. FALSE**

Rocuronium is an aminosteroid based neuromuscular blocker. It has a monoquaternary structure similar to pancuronium and vecuronium. It is much less potent with an ED 95 of 0.3 mg/kg (vec 0.056 mg/kg). The lack of potency is thought to be an important factor in determining the speed of onset of neuromuscular block. The less potent the drug, the greater the number of molecules there are available to diffuse into the NMJ. A more rapid onset is likely to be achieved with the less potent drug due to the increased diffusion gradient (due to the number of molecules) with the higher dose of the weaker agent.

Rocuronium has no active metabolites because of the lack of a methyl group at the 3 carbon position. For vecuronium the metabolite 3 disacetylvecuronium is active.

Ref: British Journal of Anaesthesia 1996; 76: 481-483

ANSWER 45

A. TRUE   B. FALSE   C. FALSE   D. TRUE   E. TRUE

Cerebral blood flow is increased by hypercapnia and hypoxia, volatile anaesthetic agents, ketamine, and hyperthermia. It is reduced with critically high ICP.

Ref: Ganong WF. Review of Medical Physiology. Lange. Ch32.

ANSWER 46

A. TRUE   B. FALSE   C. TRUE   D. TRUE   E. FALSE

Carbohydrate-rich meals have the fastest gastric emptying, protein-rich the next fastest and fatty meals the slowest gastric emptying. The entero-gastric reflex causes a reduction in gastric motility secondary to protein-rich food and hydrogen ions bathing the duodenal mucosa. Gastric emptying is normal if the pylorus is surgically resected, however vagotomy leads to gastric atony and stasis.

Ref: Ganong WF. Review of Medical Physiology, Lange

ANSWER 47

A. FALSE   B. FALSE   C. TRUE   D. TRUE   E. FALSE

The A-V O_2 difference is the difference between arterial and mixed venous O_2 content (normally ~ 5 ml O_2 / dl.) It is increased by low cardiac output states. It is decreased by poor tissue O_2 extraction eg sepsis or cyanide poisoning.

Ref: Yentis, Hirsch, Smith. Anaesthesia A to Z. Butterworth-Heinemann

ANSWER 48

A. FALSE   B. FALSE   C. TRUE   D. FALSE   E. TRUE

5-HT (serotonin) is synthesised from the amino acid precursor tryptophan derived from the diet. It is found in intestine, CNS and platelets (not neutrophils). It is metabolised by enzymes located in many tissues, including liver and brain. The measurement of urinary 5-HIAA is utilised in the diagnosis of carcinoid syndrome. There are currently at least 4 subdivisions of receptor described. The 5-HT1 receptor has been subdivided into types A, B, C, and D. Ondansetron acts on the 5-HT3 receptor. 5-HT effects on coronary vasculature depend on the concentration and type of receptor present.

Ref: British Journal of Anaesthesia 1994: 73; 395-407

ANSWER 49

A. FALSE   B. TRUE   C. FALSE   D. FALSE   E. TRUE

The serum potassium may be raised in ARF or CRF making further rises hazardous but the magnitude of the rise is the same. Some people maintain that the susceptibility to large rises in serum potassium lasts for as long as two years!

ANSWER 50

A. FALSE   B. FALSE   C. FALSE   D. FALSE   E. FALSE

Under the international standard of colours for medical gases (ISO/R32) which is in use in the UK, oxygen cylinders are black with a white top. It is a gas in the cylinder and is filled to a pressure of 134 bar (filling ratio relates to cylinders containing liquids). The cylinder has a plastic collar around its neck to identify the date when the cylinder was last examined. There is a very real risk of explosions if oil comes into contact with oxygen or nitrous oxide. To this end the valves must never be greased. It is also advisable to open the valve momentarily before attaching it to the anaesthetic machine to remove any dust that may be in the outlet, rather than letting this enter the machine.

Ref: Davis PD, Parbrook GD, Kenny GNC. Basic Physics and Measurement in Anaesthesia, 4th edn. Butterworth-Heinemann, 1995

ANSWER 51

A. TRUE   B. TRUE   C. TRUE   D. TRUE   E. FALSE

The standard deviation is the square root of the variance and represents the variability of a population or sample. 1.96 standard deviations above and below the mean will encompass 95% of the population. A tall narrow distribution curve implies a small standard deviation from the mean. The standard error of the mean is calculated from the SD divided by the square root of the number of observations and so is less than the SD in all cases. The range is the difference between maximum and minimum observed value and is a more appropriate term to apply to non-normally distributed data.

ANSWER 52

A. TRUE   B. FALSE   C. FALSE   D. TRUE   E. TRUE

Ferritin is the principal storage form of iron in tissues. 70% body iron is in haemoglobin, 27% ferritin, 3% myoglobin. Iron is transported bound to transferrin. Absorption normally matches body losses, but with iron overload mucosal cells bind iron as ferritin and are shed.

Ref: Ganong WF. Review of Medical Physiology. Lange, Ch25

ANSWER 53

A. FALSE   B. FALSE   C. TRUE   D. TRUE   E. TRUE

It has a short plasma half life, accounting for the many slow release preparations that have been developed. It is mainly metabolised in the liver and dosage adjustments are unnecessary in renal failure. Important interactions occur with the macrolides and the quinolones (ciprofloxacin) both of which reduce theophylline clearance. Phenobarbitone induces cyt P_{450} and dose increases may be necessary.

ANSWER 54

A. TRUE   B. FALSE   C. TRUE   D. FALSE   E. FALSE

Conditions where there is a drop in peripheral vascular resistance would compromise cardiac output and represent absolute contraindications to regional blockade. Aortic stenosis and pulmonary hypertension are the most dangerous conditions in this respect. Left ventricular failure, on the other hand, may be improved by the vasodilation and reduction in afterload produced by regional block. Placenta praevia is not a contraindication unless grade 4, and even then there are some authorities who would dispute the need for general anaesthesia. Spinal surgery is not a contraindication.

Ref: May A. Epidurals for Childbirth. OUP, 1994

ANSWER 55

A. FALSE   B. TRUE   C. FALSE   D. TRUE   E. FALSE

Norketamine is about 30% as active as ketamine. It does not alter the seizure threshold but is a potent cerebral vasodilator and should not be used in patients with raised intracranial pressure. It increases both $CMRO_2$ and cerebral blood flow.

PHYSICAL:

pH 3.5-5.5, pKa 7.5, 12% albumin bound

DOSE:

1-2 mg/kg iv, 10 mg/kg im

Ref: Nimmo, Rowbotham, Smith. Anaesthesia. Blackwell

ANSWER 56

A. FALSE   B. TRUE   C. FALSE   D. FALSE   E. FALSE

LIGNOCAINE

pKa = 7.9

MWt = 234

Partition coefficient = 2.9

Protein binding = 64%

Relative potency = 1

PRILOCAINE

pKa = 7.9

MWt = 220

Partition coefficient = 0.9

Protein binding = 55%

Relative potency = 1

Partition coefficient indicates lipid solubility and as a consequence, relates to potency.

Protein binding primarily influences duration of action. pKa influences degree of ionization and therefore speed of onset.

Ref: Nunn, Utting, Brown. General Anaesthesia. Butterworths.

ANSWER 57

A. TRUE   B. TRUE   C. TRUE   D. TRUE   E. FALSE

The bioavailability of a drug is the percentage of that drug that is available in the body after administration. It is expressed as a percentage with the assumption that the intravenous administration provides 100% bioavailability. If the drug is given orally it is equal to the area under the concentration time curve divided by that for an equivalent intravenous dose. Bioavailability may be different with different pharmaceutical formulations of the same drug. Extensive first pass metabolism or poor absorption are associated with low bioavailibility.

Ref: Yentis, Hirsch, Smith. Anaesthesia A to Z. Butterworth-Heinemann

ANSWER 58

A. FALSE   B. TRUE   C. TRUE   D. FALSE   E. FALSE

Fibrinolysis is usually decreased by stress including surgery. It often follows DIC and activation involves factors XII and XI.

Ref: Yentis, Hirsch, Smith. Anaesthesia A to Z. Butterworth-Heinemann

ANSWER 59

A .TRUE   B. TRUE   C. FALSE   D. TRUE   E .FALSE

Impedance is a measure of the obstruction of a capacitor to current flow. It consists of simple resistance and a component that is inversely proportional to the frequency of the a.c. current (called the reactance). It is possible to use tissue impedance to measure any change in composition as the impedance depends on the constitution of the tissue. This has allowed its use in measurement of cardiac output, spirometry, gastric emptying and limb plethysmography. However it must be calibrated against other measurements first as it is poor at absolute measurements. It is very effective at rapidly changing relative measurements once calibrated.

Inductance is the resistance induced in a coil due to the electromagnetic force produced.

Refs: Sykes MK, Vickers MD, Hull CJ. Principles of Measurement and Monitoring in Anaesthesia and Intensive Care, 3rd edn. Blackwell Scientific Publishers, 1991

Urquhart JC, Blunt MC. The Anaesthesia Viva: Physiology, Pharmacology and Statistics, Greenwich Medical Media, 1996

ANSWER 60

A. FALSE   B. TRUE   C. FALSE   D. TRUE   E. TRUE

They act by increasing insulin release from beta cells in the pancreas. Functional absence of insulin renders them useless. Tolbutamide is extensively bound to plasma proteins and displacement by such drugs as the oral anticoagulants may precipitate hypoglycaemia. The biguanide class of oral hypoglycaemic agents may cause lactic acidosis.

ANSWER 61

A. FALSE   B. TRUE   C.TRUE   D. FALSE   E. TRUE

The aetiology of shivering remains unknown but is certainly not due to volatile agents. Peroperative cooling and selective transmission of cold sensation because of a differential neural block are possible contributing factors. A small dose of pethidine may abolish it. Doxapram has also been used. Basal metabolic rate can increase 10-fold and hypoxia is common due to increased oxygen requirements for heat production.

Ref: Crossley AWA. Anaesthesia 1992;47:193

ANSWER 62

A. TRUE   B. FALSE   C. TRUE   D. TRUE   E. TRUE

The SI units consists of the seven basic units, the derived units and three units specially authorised for retention. The basic units include the candela, the derived units include the ohm and the three extra units are the litre (which could be defined in terms of dm^3 or m^3) the bar (= 105 kPa) and the metric ton. We continue to use mmHg (and cmH_2O) and atmosphere (atm) although they are non-SI units

Ref: Sykes MK, Vickers MD, Hull CJ. Principles of Measurement and Monitoring in Anaesthesia and Intensive Care, 3rd edn. Blackwell Scientific Publishers, 1991

ANSWER   63

A. TRUE   B. FALSE   C .FALSE   D. FALSE   E. TRUE

Cervical sympathetic lesions cause enophthalmos, meiosis, partial ptosis, anhydrosis and nasal mucosal engorgement.

Ref: Yentis, Hirsch, Smith. Anaesthesia A to Z. Butterworth-Heinemann

ANSWER   64

A. FALSE   B. TRUE   C. FALSE   D. TRUE   E. TRUE

The RMP of myocardial cells is -90 mV but of pacemaker cells is higher at about -60 mV. Individual myocardial cells are separated by membranes but they possess gap junctions thus allowing spread of excitation.

Ref: Ganong WF. Review of Medical Physiology. Lange.

ANSWER   65

A. FALSE   B. TRUE   C. FALSE   D. FALSE   E. TRUE

Delta waves on the EEG are abnormal 4Hz waves. They can be normal in children and during sleep. Alpha waves are prominent on closing the eyes or with increased cortical activity and beta waves prominent over the frontal area.

Ref: Yentis, Hirsch, Smith. Anaesthesia A toZ. Butterworth-Heinemann

ANSWER   66

A. TRUE   B. FALSE   C. TRUE   D. TRUE   E. TRUE

Osmolarity = the concentration (mass/volume) of osmotically active particles and is therefore volume (and temperature) dependent. Osmolality = osmoles/kgH2O. Physiological dead space = anatomical dead space + alveolar dead space. Clearance of osmoles is the amount of water necessary to excrete the osmotic load in a urine that is isotonic with plasma.

Ref: Ganong WF. Review of Medical Physiology. Lange, Ch1.

ANSWER   67

A. TRUE   B. TRUE   C. TRUE   D. TRUE   E. FALSE

Hypo- or hyper-thyroidism may occur at higher doses. Pulmonary fibrosis. if treated early and the amiodarone stopped, may regress. Corneal microdeposits rather than optic atrophy occur in long term use.

Ref: Opie L. Drugs for the Heart. Saunders

ANSWER   68

A. TRUE   B. FALSE   C. TRUE   D. FALSE   E. FALSE

Soda lime is used to absorb carbon dioxide in circle systems. 1 kg will absorb 250 litres of carbon dioxide. The granules are carefully sized in order to maximise the surface area whilst minimising the resistance to gas flow, 4-8 mesh size is most commonly used. The dust produced if the granules are crushed or disintegrate is caustic and highly irritant (causing many problems when Waters canisters were used with the canister very close to the patient). Phenolphthalein is occasionally used as an indicator and is white when fresh (alkaline) and pink when exhausted (acid). A hot canister of soda lime may indicate efficient carbon dioxide absorption, but also may be due to residual heat within the canister long after the soda lime has become exhausted.

Ref: Dorsch JA, Dorsch SE. Understanding Anesthesia Equipment; Construction, Care and Complications, 2nd edn. Williams & Wilkins, 1984

ANSWER 69

A. TRUE   B. TRUE   C. TRUE   D. TRUE   E. TRUE

Oestradiol tends to cause retention of salt and water in the kidneys and locally (hence its inclusion in cosmetic creams designed to reduce wrinkles by provoking mild local oedema). On the other hand, progesterone inhibits aldosterone which will tend to increase NaCl excretion.

Ref: Despopoulos A, Silbernagl S. Color Atlas of Physiology, 232-271

ANSWER 70

A. FALSE   B. FALSE   C. TRUE   D. TRUE   E. TRUE

Patient heat loss is mainly due to radiation (40-50%) and, to a lesser extent, convection (defined as in the question) and evaporation. About 15% of heat loss in the anaesthetised patient is via the respiratory tract. The main part of this is due to the latent heat needed to vaporise water to humidify the gas within the trachea. This can be minimised by humidification. Warming equipment such as electric blankets and water-filled mattresses have caused thermal burns in anaesthetised patients. The risk of burns is greater if there is poor blood supply as blood can help conduct the heat away from the site of potential injury.

Ref: Davis PD, Parbrook GD, Kenny GNC. Basic Physics and Measurement in Anaesthesia, 4th edn. Butterworth-Heinemann, 1995

ANSWER 71

A. FALSE   B. TRUE   C. TRUE   D. FALSE   E. FALSE

Salt deficit leads initially to a decrease in ADH secretion, otherwise renin, angiotensin and aldosterone levels rise as stated. Osmolality is measured in milliosmoles/kg H_2O. ADH is secreted by the posterior pituitary.

Ref: Despopoulos A, Silbernagl S. Color Atlas of Physiology, 120-152

ANSWER 72

A. FALSE   B. FALSE   C. FALSE   D. TRUE   E. FALSE

NCEPOD is an audit project and deals with postoperative deaths within 30 days of surgery. Each hospital has a nominated reporting officer, who is usually a pathologist. Only a sample of cases (1 in 5 reported) is taken and dealt with in detail. A large number of forms are never completed and this is a major deficiency, as the most reprehensible cases are probably never reported.

ANSWER 73

A. FALSE   B. TRUE   C. TRUE   D. TRUE   E. FALSE

Blood loss in ml is normally-distributed interval scale data and the Mann–Whitney test is used for analysis of ordinal data. The Chi-squared test measures differences between nominal data, which is usually yes/no, survival/death. ANOVA is analysis of variance and compares normally-distributed interval scale data in multiple groups. It is fearsomely complicated. The t-test is used when dealing with normally-distributed interval scale data. Baldness is not interval scale data.

ANSWER 74

A. FALSE   B. FALSE   C. FALSE   D. TRUE   E. FALSE

Riva-Rocci first described using occlusion to measure blood pressure in 1896. Korotkoff then described the use of auscultation in 1905: The systolic pressure is taken as the first time the sounds are heard as the cuff is deflated from a supra-systolic pressure. There may then be muffling and resurgence of the sounds (Korotkoff's second and third phase) before the sudden muffing of the sound (fourth phase) and then silence (fifth phase). The latter two are both taken as diastolic pressures, though both are actually above the pressure recorded directly. The cuff should be 20% greater than the diameter of the arm. A mercury sphygmomanometer measures pressure above atmospheric ('gauge' pressure) and as such has air in the space above the mercury column (otherwise there would be a column of mercury 760 mm high before the cuff were connected to the patient).

Ref: Parbrook GD, Gray WM. The measurement of blood pressure. In: Scurr C, Feldman S, Soni N (Eds) Scientific Foundations of Anaesthesia; The Basis of Intensive Care, 4th edn. Heinemann Medical Books, 1990, pp 70-81

ANSWER 75

A. FALSE   B. TRUE   C. TRUE   D. TRUE   E. FALSE

The train of four is the most common method of monitoring neuromuscular blockade in theatre. It consists of four supramaximal twitches at 0.5 sec intervals (2 Hz). Non-depolarising blockade is characterised by fade (where the strength of the twitches decreases from first (T1) to the last (T4)), and post-tetanic facilitation. Fade is believed to be due to inadequacy of presynaptic ACh release in response to rapid stimulation and post-tetanic facilitation is due to accumulation of ACh in the synaptic cleft following tetanic stimulation. The facial nerve is often used for monitoring because it is convenient. Its response to muscle relaxants is similar to that of the diaphragm although it tends to be obscured by direct muscle stimulation.

A patient should show at least 70% recovery of T4 before he is suitable for extubation rather than merely its presence.

Ref: Silverman DG, Brull SJ. Monitoring neuromuscular block. In: Sanford TJ (Ed) Clinical Issues in Monitoring. W.B. Saunders, 1994, pp 237-260

ANSWER 76

A. FALSE   B. FALSE   C. TRUE   D. TRUE   E. FALSE

The femoral vein lies just medial to the pulsation of the femoral artery; when cannulating the internal jugular, it is the ipsilateral nipple that represents the target. The thoracic duct lies on the left and is relatively safe when the right-sided approach is used. The Seldinger technique involves the passage of a cannula over a guide wire previously inserted through a needle. Pneumothorax is a hazard of any central cannulation technique in the upper body, but especially the subclavian approach.

Ref:(no reference)

ANSWER 77

A. FALSE   B. TRUE   C. FALSE   D. FALSE   E. FALSE

Monosynaptic reflexes generally originate and terminate in the same muscle and are very fast (typically 20 ms). Polysynaptic reflexes include the protective reflexes, nutritional reflexes (swallowing, sucking), locomotion reflexes and vegetative reflexes (circulation, respiration, sex, bladder etc).

Ref: Despopoulos A, Silbernagl S. Color Atlas of Physiology. 272-325

ANSWER 78

A. FALSE   B. TRUE   C. TRUE   D. FALSE   E. TRUE

The Mapleson classification of breathing systems has six classifications A-F. The Lack circuit and the Magill attachment are examples of Mapleson A systems. They are very efficient for spontaneous breathing (requiring a fresh gas flow (FGF) equal to alveolar ventilation - less than minute ventilation (MV)). They are much less efficient for controlled ventilation (FGF = 3 x MV). The Mapleson D (including the coaxial Bain circuit) is most efficient for controlled ventilation. The Bain circuit requires a FGF of 70 ml/kg to maintain normocarbia. The Mapleson F (Jackson-Rees) is a modification of the Ayre's T-piece (Mapleson E) designed to minimise resistance to gas flow and ideal for paediatric use

Ref: Faust RJ (ed) Anesthesiology Review, 2nd edn. Churchill Livingstone, 1994

ANSWER 79

A. TRUE   B. FALSE   C. TRUE   D. TRUE   E. FALSE

The normal process is de-acetylation which becomes saturated. Hypokalaemia is usual.

Ref: British Journal of Anaesthesia 1993; 70(5): 562

ANSWER 80

A. TRUE   B. FALSE   C. TRUE   D. FALSE   E. FALSE

Midazolam is a water soluble benzodiazepine which unlike diazepam does not require formulating in a solubilising agent. At a pH of less than 4 the imidazole ring is open. At physiological pH the ring closes, conferring lipid solubility. It is almost completely broken down by hydroxylation in the liver to the active metabolites 1- and 4-hydroxy-midazolam.

PHYSICAL:

>90% protein bound, Vd 0.8-1.5 l/kg

ANSWER 81

A. TRUE   B. FALSE   C. FALSE   D. FALSE   E. FALSE

Mivacurium chloride is presented as an aqueous solution which is acidic, the pH being maintained in the range 3.5-5.0 by the addition of hydrochloric acid. It has a shelf-life of 18 months when stored below 25 degrees C. It is a non-depolarising neuromuscular blocker which undergoes hydrolysis by plasma cholinesterase. Patients with defective or reduced levels of this enzyme may therefore undergo prolonged neuromuscular block. It is a short-acting benzyl-isoquinolinium compound but is a non depolarising agent.

ANSWER 82

A. TRUE   B. FALSE   C. TRUE   D. TRUE   E. TRUE

The knee jerk reflex describes contraction of the quadriceps in response to stretch of the patellar tendon. The sensory organ is the muscle spindle, which when stretched sends signals to the CNS where the single synapse (glutamate) occurs with the motor supply to the muscle. In addition the Ia fibre from the muscle spindle synapses with an inhibitory interneurone (golgi bottle neurone) which releases inhibitory glycine at the motor neurone to the antagonistic muscle - so called reciprocal innervation. The knee jerk reflex involves the nerve roots L2,3,4.

Ref: Ganong WF. Review of Medical Physiology. Lange.

ANSWER 83

A. TRUE   B. FALSE   C. FALSE   D. TRUE   E. FALSE

These were implemented to reduce malpractice premiums but have become accepted as the basis of good anaesthetic practice since then. They are:

1. Presence of the anaesthetist (not assistant) throughout procedure and until patient fully recovered.
2. ECG.
3. Blood pressure and heart rate measured and recorded every 5 minutes.
4. Observation of ventilation: Movement of the bag, or monitoring breath sounds, or end-tidal CO_2.
5. Observation of the circulation: Palpation of pulse, or SpO_2, although this is not a specific requirement.
6. Disconnection alarm.
7. Measurement of FiO_2. The ability to record patient temperature was added as a footnote.

Ref: Nunn, Utting, Burnell Brown. General Anaesthesia. Butterworth-Heinemann

ANSWER 84

A. FALSE   B. FALSE   C. TRUE   D. FALSE   E. TRUE

The trigeminal nerve (V) supplies the muscles of mastication (but not the tongue, which is mostly hypoglossal except for palatoglossus which is vagally innervated) and sensation to the forehead and face in the distribution ophthalmic, maxillary and mandibular branches. This includes sensation from the cornea. VII provides motor supply to the muscles of facial expression (including orbicularis oculi, required for the efferent limb of the corneal reflex). Taste sensation to the posterior third of the tongue is provided by the glossopharyngeal (IX), the rest being supplied by the chorda tympani accompanying the facial nerve (VII).

Ref: Yentis, Hirsch, Smith. Anaesthesia A to Z. Butterworth-Heinemann

ANSWER 85

A. TRUE   B. FALSE   C. TRUE   D. TRUE   E. TRUE

Generally, the parasympathetic supply to the GUT is via pre-ganglionic vagal fibres, which cause increased activity in intestinal smooth muscle. The sympathetic supply is post-ganglionic, but may end on cholinergic neurones or on smooth muscle fibres directly.

Ref: Ganong WF. Review of Medical Physiology, Lange

ANSWER 86

A. TRUE   B. TRUE   C. FALSE   D. TRUE   E. FALSE

In the lateral position, the lower dome of the diaphragm is pushed higher in the chest and therefore contracts more effectively. Both V and Q are higher in the dependent lung but Q is relatively greater than V, hence V/Q < 1, PO_2 is lower and PCO_2 is higher in the dependent areas.

Ref: Nunn JF. Applied Respiratory Physiology. Butterworth-Heinemann

ANSWER 87

A. TRUE   B. FALSE   C. TRUE   D. FALSE   E. TRUE

Liver blood flow in the adult would normally be c1500 ml/min, 70% volume via the portal vein. Portal and hepatic flow converges at the sinusoids before common drainage to the central lobular veins. Supply is largely pressure dependent but in the hypovolaemic patient noradrenergic vasoconstriction of the hepatic arterioles occurs.

Ref: Ganong WF. Review of Medical Physiology. Lange. Ch32

ANSWER 88

A. FALSE   B. FALSE   C. TRUE   D. FALSE   E. FALSE

The ASA classification does not predict outcome; it indicates preoperative status and suggests the degree of skill required to deal with the case. It is widely used in audit to indicate the severity of disease and in research to standardise patients. The Harvard Minimum Monitoring Standards were developed as a result of escalating malpractice premiums. E indicates emergency, but has a different definition from that used in the Confidential Enquiries into Perioperative Death.

The ASA classes are, briefly:

I: Fit and well

II: Mild systemic disease

III: Disease restricting activity

IV: Severe systemic disease which is a constant threat to life

V: Moribund and not expected to survive 24 hours.

ANSWER 89

A. TRUE   B. FALSE   C. TRUE   D. FALSE   E. TRUE

Dantrolene can be given intravenously, orally or intra-muscularly (if no other route is available). The initial dose is 1 mg/kg , repeated up to 10 mg/kg. It can cause respiratory failure secondary to skeletal muscle weakness. It causes relaxation by a direct action on excitation–contraction coupling.

PHYSICAL:

pH 9.5, 80-90% protein bound

DOSE:

1-10 mg/kg, ampoules contain 20 mg dantrolene, 3 g mannitol, NaOH.

ANSWER 90

A. TRUE   B. FALSE   C. TRUE   D. FALSE   E. TRUE

Renal clearance = Urine drug conc./Plasma drug conc. x Urine flow rateIf a drug is filtered and not reabsorbed nor secreted, its renal clearance is 120 ml/min (ie GFR). A drug that is secreted actively such that it is cleared completely in one passage through the kidney has a clearance that approximates to renal plasma flow (750 ml/min). A lipophilic drug is absorbed passively as it passes through the nephron so that the final urine concentration equilibrates to plasma concentration and therefore its clearance = urine flow rate x 1.

Ref: Nimmo, Rowbotham, Smith. Anaesthesia, Blackwell, chapter 15

Exam 2

QUESTION 1

Regarding diet and metabolism

- **A.** Folic acid is an essential amino acid.
- **B.** 1 kilojoule = 4.2 kilocalories.
- **C.** A minimum daily protein intake of 0.5 g/kg bodyweight is required to match basal losses.
- **D.** Increase in fat intake will cause a fall in the respiratory quotient.
- **E.** Fat is not required in the adult diet.

QUESTION 2

Electric shocks (with a 240 V main supply)

- **A.** A sustained current of approximately 15–50 mA flowing from one hand to the other will probably lead to death due to asphyxiation.
- **B.** A current of 1–2 mA flowing from one hand to the other will be felt as a tingling sensation.
- **C.** Are made safer if the patient is earthed.
- **D.** Currents of greater than 5 A flowing from one hand to the other will cause myocardial stand-still.
- **E.** A residual current circuit breaker improves safety by switching off the supply when the current flow at the Live and Neutral conductors differs.

QUESTION 3

Nerve stimulators

- **A.** Double burst is of particular value in assessing blockade when there is no response to the train-of-four.
- **B.** A fading pattern to the train-of-four excludes prolonged action of suxamethonium
- **C.** When used to locate nerves for regional blockade the positive electrode should be attached to the locating needle.
- **D.** The post tetanic count is particularly useful for assessing the patient's suitability for extubation.
- **E.** The ideal nerve for neuromuscular blockade assessment is generally considered to be the facial nerve.

QUESTION 4

In a nitrous oxide cylinder

A. The filling ratio is the volume of N_2O divided by the volume of the cylinder
B. A filling ratio of 0.67 is normal in temperate countries
C. The pressure in the full cylinder is 134 bar
D. The critical temperature of the N_2O is higher than room temperature
E. The cylinder is painted blue with white and blue quartered shoulders

QUESTION 5 ·

In a normal adult male

A. Alveolar minute ventilation at rest = 4 to 5 litres
B. A maximum breathing capacity or voluntary minute ventilation of 150 litres would be considered normal
C. Vital capacity is equivalent to the inspiratory capacity plus functional residual capacity
D. FEV_1 should be less than the functional residual capacity
E. Standard lung volumes may be corrected to 0 degrees Celsius and 760 mmHg using dry air (ATPS)

QUESTION 6

Concerning nerve conduction

A. A-delta fibres are the slowest as they are unmyelinated
B. A-beta fibres exhibit saltatory conduction
C. C fibres are unmyelinated
D. A-alpha fibres conduct at 70-120 m/s
E. A-gamma fibres are sensory to muscle spindles.

QUESTION 7

At high altitudes the following occur

A. When breathing air at 2000 m, ventilation is driven predominantly by PaO_2
B. Above 7000 m a climber breathing air is likely to become unconsciou
C. It is not possible to achieve a PaO_2 of 13 kPa at altitudes where atmospheric pressure is less than 25 kPa
D. Acute compensation mechanisms include an increase in erythropoietin levels
E. Increased bicarbonate excretion occurs.

QUESTION 8

Ephedrine

A. Is a catecholamine
B. Acts both directly and indirectly on adrenergic receptors
C. Elevates the blood pressure for about the same duration as adrenaline when given in equipotent doses
D. Exhibits tachyphylaxis
E. Can be given orally

QUESTION 9

Concerning heparin

A. It is a water soluble organic acid
B. After intravenous injection, the onset of anticoagulant effect is about 30 minutes
C. It crosses the placenta in significant amounts after maternal administration
D. It has a prolonged duration of action in the presence of liver dysfunction
E. Is metabolised by heparinase to metabolites which are pharmacologically active

QUESTION 10

Concerning direct measurement of arterial blood pressure

A. The diastolic pressure will be underestimated in a resonant system
B. Air bubbles in the tubing will not affect the measured mean pressure
C. The transducer should be placed level with the patient's posterior axillary line
D. The diastolic pressure will be underestimated in a damped system
E. Information concerning the systemic vascular resistance can be obtained

QUESTION 11

2 litre reservoir bags

A. Are made from carbon-impregnated rubber
B. Are antistatic
C. Hold 2 litres when fully distended
D. Are designed to allow the internal pressure to reach no more than 80 cmH$_2$O
E. Often have a loop on the end in order to help drying after cleaning

QUESTION 12

On tilting a patient from supine to vertical

A. Reduced renin secretion occurs
B. Cerebral vascular resistance is reduced
C. Cerebral blood flow falls by 40%
D. Cardiac output is reduced
E. The R-R interval shortens

QUESTION 13

The following drugs enhance the action of warfarin

A. Cholestyramine
B. Cimetidine
C. Phenobarbitone
D. Rifampicin
E. Tricyclic antidepressants

QUESTION 14

The following drugs preferentially act at alpha-1 adrenoceptors

A. Phenylephrine
B. Clonidine
C. Naphazoline
D. Methoxamine
E. Alpha-methylnoradrenaline

QUESTION 15

Regarding first order kinetics

A. The rate constant is the time taken for concentration to fall by 50%
B. Concentration declines exponentially
C. Time constant = 1 / Rate constant
D. Half life = 3 time constants
E. Rate of elimination is proportional to concentration

QUESTION 16

The odds ratio

A. May be used to compare the starting prices of two racehorses
B. Deals with exposure and outcome
C. Estimates risk of an outcome
D. An odds ratio of 2 would suggest double the risk of developing a carcinoma following exposure to the carcinogen
E. Defines the correlation between statistical outcome and clinical outcome

QUESTION 17

Concerning statistical analysis of data

A. The null hypothesis describes the probability that a relationship exists between two samples
B. Descriptive statistics produce mean, median and mode from data
C. Analytical statistics are the same as inferential statistics
D. The mode is the measurement which lies exactly between each end of a range of values ranked in order
E. Skewed data invalidates further statistical analysis

QUESTION 18

The following statements concerning colloids are true

A. Hydroxyethyl starch is produced from cattle bone
B. Dextrans are produced by bacteria grown in a sucrose medium
C. In therapeutic volumes, dextran 40 interferes with haemostasis
D. The gelatin Haemaccel has a mean molecular weight of 450,000
E. The intravascular half-life of hydroxyethyl starch is less than 24 hours

QUESTION 19

The following are examples of pharmacokinetic drug interactions

A. Lithium and thiazide diuretics
B. Digoxin and amiodarone
C. Phenytoin and cimetidine
D. Beta blockers and verapamil
E. Ethanol and diazepam

QUESTION 20

Concerning phaeochromocytoma

A. The condition may present with refractory hypertension
B. Elevated urinary vanillyl-mandelic acid levels may indicate the diagnosis
C. Propranolol may be used initially to control the condition
D. Hypertension after completion of surgery and removal of the tumour is rare
E. Steroid replacement therapy will be needed

QUESTION 21

The following are indications for the use of ACE inhibitors

A. Hypertension in pregnancy
B. Essential hypertension
C. Hypertension secondary to bilateral renal artery stenosis
D. Following acute myocardial infarction
E. In severe heart failure

QUESTION 22

Transport processes in the kidney include

A. Tubular secretion of NH_3 in both proximal and distal tubules
B. Glomerular filtration of all molecules under 5 nm diameter
C. Reabsorption of proteins by pinocytosis
D. Reabsorption of 160 g glucose per day
E. Excretion of bicarbonate ions buffered by phosphate

QUESTION 23

A Clark electrode

A. Has a silver/silver chloride cathode
B. Has a copper electrode
C. Has an electrolyte medium of aluminium hydroxide
D. Requires a battery
E. Relies on a similar reaction to one within the mitochondrion

QUESTION 24

The sinoatrial node pacemaker cell action potential

A. Has a longer plateau phase following vagal stimulation
B. Has a normal threshold potential of +20 mV
C. Has a more negative maximum diastolic potential following vagal stimulation
D. Has a steeper prepotential slope following sympathetic stimulation
E. Has a shorter duration in the presence of hypothermia

QUESTION 25

Ondansetron

A. Can only be administered intravenously
B. Has a plasma half-life of 8 hours
C. Is metabolised by hydroxylation in the liver
D. May produce constipation, headache and flushing
E. Is a 5HT-3 agonist

QUESTION 26

Mivacurium chloride

A. Is a mixture of three stereo-isomers in approximately equal proportions
B. Has a prolonged duration of action in patients with severe liver disease
C. Can cause significant release of histamine
D. Can be associated with facial erythema, tachycardia and hypotension
E. Has no effect on autonomic ganglia at clinical doses

QUESTION 27

Carbon dioxide

A. Freely diffuses across the blood : brain barrier
B. Has a solubility coefficient of 0.225 mmol/l/mmHg
C. Gives rise to the same pH change in CSF as it does in blood
D. Transport by haemoglobin is inhibited by rising oxygen saturation
E. Has direct sympathomimetic activity

QUESTION 28

Skeletal muscle

A. Has a resting membrane potential of -90 mV
B. Has an absolute refractory period of about 200 ms
C. Has thin filaments composed of actin and myosin chains
D. A-bands shorten during muscle contraction
E. Contraction is initiated by calcium binding to calmodulin

QUESTION 29

Iron absorption is dependent on

A. Total body vitamin C
B. HCl in the stomach
C. An intact colonic mucosa
D. Total body iron
E. Erythropoietin levels in the blood

QUESTION 30

The following are side effects of thiazide diuretics

A. Hyperuricaemia
B. Hyponatraemia
C. Hyperglycaemia
D. Hypokalaemic, hypochloraemic acidosis
E. Hypocalcaemia

QUESTION 31

Flow through a tube

A. If the Reynolds number is high (>2500) flow is likely to be laminar
B. In laminar flow the peak velocity is twice the average velocity
C. Turbulent flow is likely at the connection between the endotracheal tube and the anaesthetic circuit
D. Switching from oxygen to helium significantly improves laminar flow
E. The velocity at which transition between turbulent and laminar flow occurs is called the critical velocity

QUESTION 32

During production of thyroid hormones

A. TSH secretion is modified by direct negative feedback of T3 and T4 on the pituitary
B. Increased thyroid activity is marked by abundance of colloid
C. D-Thyroxine has only a small fraction of the activity of L-thyroxine
D. Thyroxine is also formed by peripheral conversion of T3
E. About 85% of circulating thyroid hormones remain bound to thyroglobulin

QUESTION 33

Glucagon release

A. Stimulates gluconeogenesis
B. Inhibits adenylate cyclase in liver cells
C. Stimulates secretion of growth hormone
D. Is inhibited by cortisol
E. Is stimulated by theophylline

QUESTION 34

Gentamicin

A. Is poorly lipid soluble
B. Inhibits protein synthesis in bacterial ribosomes
C. Is transported across bacterial cell membranes by an oxygen-dependent active transport system
D. Is excreted exclusively by the kidney
E. Inhibits the effects of neuromuscular blocking agents

QUESTION 35

Enalapril

A. Is a prodrug
B. Is 90% protein bound
C. Contains a sulphydryl group
D. Is largely excreted by the kidney
E. Is not thought to scavenge free radicals

QUESTION 36

Parathyroid hormone

A. Causes osteoclast activation
B. Is a peptide
C. Has direct activity on the intestine
D. Decreases phosphate excretion
E. Stimulates 25-hydroxylation of cholecalciferol

QUESTION 37

Nifedipine

A. Has a structure similar to verapamil
B. Is absorbed more rapidly when given sublingually compared to intranasally
C. Undergoes extensive first pass metabolism in the liver
D. Is metabolised to inert products
E. Has a significant effect on the AV node

QUESTION 38

Dystrophica myotonica

A. Is an inherited condition with autosomal dominant transmission
B. Is associated with frontal balding, diabetes, cataracts and retardation
C. Is exacerbated by heat and exertion
D. May be treated with procyclidine
E. Neostigmine, if used in the reversal of non-depolarising neuromuscular blockade, causes prolonged weakness

QUESTION 39

Fibreoptic tracheal intubation

A. Uses technology based on 20 micrometer diameter glass fibres in bundles
B. Is best performed by the oral route
C. Cocaine paste 10% applied to the nasal mucosa reduces the incidence of haemorrhage and improves the view
D. Krausse's forceps are used to block the superior laryngeal nerve in the piriform fossa
E. Can be performed with the cervical spine immobilised in a rigid collar

QUESTION 40

Pancreatic juice

A. Is acidic
B. Is bicarbonate ion rich
C. Contains trypsinogen
D. Secretion is reduced with increased vagal tone
E. Approximately 1500 ml are secreted per day in a healthy adult

QUESTION 41

Blood flow (ml/100 g/min) in a 70 kg man

A. To the liver and brain are approximately equivalent
B. Is about 420 to the kidneys
C. Is greater to the brain than the heart
D. Is higher to skeletal muscle than to the skin
E. Is about 45 to the skin

QUESTION 42

Porphyria

A. Can be induced by alcohol, pregnancy and muscular activity
B. Is characterised by the induction of the enzyme d-aminolaevulinic acid synthetase
C. Anaesthesia does not induce the erythropoetic forms of the disease
D. The use of tourniquets is contraindicated
E. Barbiturate anaesthesia must be avoided

QUESTION 43

Correlation coefficient

A. Is usually denoted by the symbol "c"
B. Is measured on a scale of 0 to 1
C. A positive value implies that a rise in one variable accompanies a rise in the other
D. Describes the degree of association between two variables
E. Describes the degree of agreement between two variables

QUESTION 44

Edrophonium

A. Has a more rapid onset than neostigmine
B. Is more potent than neostigmine
C. Is eliminated largely by the kidney
D. Is lipid soluble and can be given orally in the treatment of myasthenia gravis
E. Inhibits plasma cholinesterase in addition to acetylcholinesterase

QUESTION 45

Etomidate

A. Is a carboxylated imidazole-containing compound
B. Is poorly water soluble at acidic pH, and lipid soluble at physiological pH
C. Produces post-operative nausea and vomiting more frequently than thiopentone
D. Is almost completely hydrolysed to an inactive metabolite by hepatic microsomal enzymes
E. Causes involuntary movements more frequently than it causes pain following intravenous injection

QUESTION 46

The neuroleptic malignant syndrome

A. Can be precipitated by droperidol
B. Is potentially fatal
C. Is characterised by dystonia, rigidity and hypothermia
D. Can result in autonomic lability
E. May lead to rhabdomyolysis

QUESTION 47

Intra-pleural pressure

A. Can be measured with an oesophageal ballon
B. Is related to diffusion of O_2 into the inter-pleural space
C. Becomes increasingly negative with increasing lung volumes during inspiration
D. Equals atmospheric pressure at FRC
E. Is higher in the dependent parts of the lung

QUESTION 48

Atracurium

A. Releases histamine
B. Is suitable for use in anephric patients
C. Is metabolised by ester hydrolysis
D. Some of its metabolites have neuromuscular blocking activity
E. Has an increased volume of distribution in cirrhotic patients

QUESTION 49

The Confidential Enquiries into Maternal Deaths (CEMD)

A. Does not include data from Scotland
B. Is the longest-running medical audit project in the world
C. Reports every three years
D. Deals with maternal death during pregnancy and up to 42 days post delivery or termination
E. Continues to identify haemorrhage as the commonest cause of death

QUESTION 50

Ciprofloxacin

A. Is a monobactam
B. Is useful in the treatment of infection with Gram negative bacteria
C. Has reliable activity against Gram positive organisms
D. Can only be given intravenously
E. Dose not require dose reductions in renal failure.

QUESTION 51

Concerning desflurane

A. It is a chlorinated methyl ethyl ether
B. It has a boiling point approximately the same as that of isoflurane
C. It has a molecular weight which is the same as that of enflurane
D. It is stable in soda lime
E. About 0.2% is recoverable as metabolite

QUESTION 52

The following statements about suxamethonium are true

A. It is the muscle relaxant most frequently implicated in allergic reactions
B. It is metabolised to two molecules of acetylcholine by the action of plasma pseudocholinesterase
C. The rise in intraocular pressure caused by its administration lasts for up to half an hour
D. It may cause a bradycardia due to stimulation of nicotinic receptors
E. The Phase II block seen after repeated administration or infusion is reliably reversed using neostigmine

QUESTION 53

Cardiac muscle can utilize the following energy substrates

A. Carbohydrate
B. Ketones
C. Amino acids
D. Free fatty acids
E. Pyruvic acid

QUESTION 54

Concerning the cardiac cycle

A. Aortic pressure is highest at the end of ventricular systole
B. Left atrial pressure is highest during left ventricular systole
C. Aortic blood flow is lowest at the end of diastole
D. Aortic pressure exceeds left ventricular pressure late in systole
E. A fourth heart sound, if present, will be heard during atrial systole

QUESTION 55

Concerning white blood cells

A. The average half-life in the circulation of neutrophils is 6 hours
B. Lymphocytes are produced in the spleen
C. Basophils contain heparin and histamine and are phagocytic
D. Neutrophils attack parasites
E. T lymphocytes originate in the thyroid

QUESTION 56

The following ions have an intracellular concentration that is at least twice their normal plasma concentration

A. Potassium
B. Magnesium
C. Chloride
D. Bicarbonate
E. Phosphate

QUESTION 57

When assessing the airway preoperatively

A. The Mallampati grading accurately predicts difficult intubation
B. Mallampati grade 4 indicates a view of the soft palate
C. Wilson grade C accurately predicts difficult intubation
D. The ability to put chin on chest is a reliable indication of ease of intubation
E. Vertebro-basilar insufficiency may be detected

QUESTION 58

Measurement of respiratory nitrogen concentration

A. Is a valuable method of detecting air emboli in neurosurgery
B. May be performed by infra-red absorption spectroscopy
C. May be performed by Raman scattering
D. A rapid fall in the early stages of general anaesthesia suggests a leak in the circuit
E. May be valuable to ensure adequacy of pre-oxygenation

QUESTION 59

The Glasgow Coma Scale

A. Indicates the severity of head injur

B. May be used as a prognostic guide

C. A score of 2 is incompatible with survival

D. If the patient's best motor response is flexion to pain, this scores 3 points

E. Was first described by Dr Fergus Glasgow in 1973

QUESTION 60

Tricyclic antidepressants

A. Have rapid onset of action

B. May cause a dry mouth and blurred vision

C. May cause tachycardia

D. Do not produce postural hypotension

E. Inhibit neuronal uptake of noradrenaline

QUESTION 61

In pulse oximetry

A. The SpO_2 is determined by the absorbance of light of wavelengths 660nm and 940nm

B. Methaemoglobin causes the SpO_2 to approach 85%

C. Oxyhaemoglobin absorbs better at the longer wavelength

D. Fetal haemoglobin gives an inaccurately high reading of saturation

E. The machine is less accurate at low rather than high saturations

QUESTION 62

During vomiting

A. Afferents may arise from the limbic system

B. Motor efferent activity is initiated by cells in the lateral wall of the 3rd ventricle

C. Reverse peristalsis occurs in the duodenum

D. The glottis opens

E. The breath is held in full inspiration

QUESTION 63

Surgical diathermy

A. Produces current with a frequency of 100 Hz

B. Must always be earthed

C. Should never be used in patients with pacemakers

D. May cause explosions even when non-flammable anaesthetic agents are in use

E. May cause burns under ECG electrodes

QUESTION   64

The oxygen failure warning device

A. Is only required on anaesthesia machines if there is no oxygen concentration analyser
B. Must last for at least 15 seconds
C. Should be powered by a battery or the gas supply
D. Should cut off the fresh gas supply as soon as the oxygen pressure starts to fail
E. May only be switched off temporarily before the oxygen supply is reconnected

QUESTION   65

The following drugs cross the placenta rapidly

A. Atropine
B. Neostigmine
C. Metoclopramide
D. Ketamine
E. Diazepam

QUESTION   66

Concerning the visual pathway

A. Optic tract lesions will cause a bitemporal hemianopia
B. Optic chiasma lesions will cause a homonymous hemianopia
C. Occipital lesions may spare the macula
D. Optic nerve lesions will cause unilateral loss of vision
E. Lesions of the geniculocalcarine tract will cause a central scotoma

QUESTION   67

The following potentiate the action of non–depolarising neuromuscular blockers

A. Diethyl ether
B. Quinidine
C. Enflurane
D. Lithium
E. Dantrolene

QUESTION   68

Regarding CSF

A. Formation is largely independent of ICP
B. Removal is increased as ICP rises
C. It is secreted by the arachnoid villi
D. It leaves the IVth ventricle via the foramina of Monro
E. A potassium ion concentration of 3 mmol/l is normal

QUESTION 69

The normal electrocardiogram

A. Between the T wave and the next P wave the myocardial potential is zero
B. Repolarisation takes place in the opposite direction as depolarisation
C. The electrodes have a aluminium/saline interface
D. CM_5 is a modification of lead V_5
E. Can give good information concerning the myocardial contractility

QUESTION 70

Ropivacaine

A. Is a racaemic mixture of the S and R isomers
B. Shows an improved motor-sensory separation of local anaesthetic effects that is useful in providing pain relief
C. Has a similar pKa to Bupivacaine
D. Demonstrates similar lipid solubility to bupivacaine
E. Has a clearance that is 30% less than bupivacaine

QUESTION 71

Dantrolene

A. Is useful in the treatment of malignant hyperthermia
B. Significantly prolongs the action of non-depolarising muscle relaxants
C. Is a respiratory stimulant
D. Reduces the efflux of calcium from the sarcoplasmic reticulum in skeletal muscle
E. Is effective in the treatment of the neuroleptic malignant syndrome

QUESTION 72

Soda lime contains

A. Potassium hydroxide
B. Silica
C. Calcium hydroxide
D. Magnesium hydroxide
E. Aluminium carbonate

QUESTION 73

In recovery

A. One nurse for every two patients is acceptable
B. Spontaneously breathing patients should be transferred to recovery with oxygen by facemask
C. Oliguria is best treated by a small dose of a loop diuretic
D. Non-steroidal anti-inflammatories (NSAIDs) should not be used in patients with a history of bronchospasm
E. Dermatomal level of regional analgesia need not be recorded as long as the patient is pain-free

QUESTION 74

The following cardiovascular changes have occurred at term pregnancy in relation to pre-pregnant values

A. Cardiac output increased by 20%
B. Stroke volume increased by 50%
C. Decreased SVR
D. Increased heart rate
E. Increased mean arterial blood pressure

QUESTION 75

In sickle cell disease

A. The rate of globin synthesis is normal
B. The abnormality is caused by a mutation of thymine to adenine
C. It is generally milder in Asians than in Africans
D. Distribution parallels that of plasmodium falciparum malaria
E. HbS forms crystals when exposed to low oxygen tensions

QUESTION 76

Concerning the paediatric airway

A. Valveless breathing systems offer an advantage because room air will not be entrained
B. The appropriate tracheal tube size can be calculated using age in years
C. The limb on the Jackson-Rees modification of the Ayre's T-piece should exceed minute volume
D. Fresh gas flow must exceed 3 litres/min with the T-piece
E. The right main bronchus is more easily intubated inadvertently in the neonate than in the adult

QUESTION 77

Concerning cardiac tissue action potentials

A. The SA node action potential is mainly due to calcium ions
B. The AV node pre-potential is mainly due to sodium ions
C. Cardiac muscle repolarisation is mainly due to potassium ions
D. The SA node pre-potential lasts the longest of the pacemakers
E. Atrial muscle fibres do not possess pre-potentials

QUESTION 78

In determining the energy content of foodstuffs

A. A calorie is the amount of heat required to warm 1 g of water from 15 to 16 degrees centigrade
B. The available calorific value of carbohydrates = 4.1 kcal/g
C. The physical calorific value of protein = 4.1 kcal/g
D. The physical calorific value of fat is 9.3 kcal/g
E. A protein diet raises the metabolic rate

QUESTION 79

Respiratory insufficiency in recovery

- **A.** Should be treated with 400 mcg naloxone in the first instance
- **B.** The cause may be elucidated by the application of a nerve stimulator
- **C.** Administration of carbon dioxide is an appropriate measure if hypocarbia is the cause
- **D.** Hypokalaemia may contribute to prolonged neuromuscular blockade
- **E.** If due to the prolonged action of suxamethonium, will reverse with neostigmine 2.5 mg and glycopyrrolate 0.5 mg

QUESTION 80

Awareness under anaesthesia

- **A.** The EEG is a reliable indicator of awareness
- **B.** The incidence is about 1:50,000 anaesthetics
- **C.** The incidence is higher in obstetric surgery than general surgery
- **D.** The addition of high doses of fentanyl to a nitrous oxide/oxygen anaesthetic is effective for eliminating awareness
- **E.** Lower oesophageal contractility declines with increasing depth of anaesthesia

QUESTION 81

Concerning motor pathways

- **A.** Fibres arise from pyramidal cells in the post-central gyrus area of cerebral cortex
- **B.** The lower limbs are represented uppermost in the motor cortex
- **C.** The hands have a disproportionately small representation
- **D.** Most motor fibres decussate in the lower medulla
- **E.** Fibres in the anterior corticospinal tract remain uncrossed until their spinal level

QUESTION 82

The following are non-parametric tests

- **A.** The Mann-Whitney U test
- **B.** The Wilcoxon signed rank sum test
- **C.** The Chi-squared test
- **D.** ANOVA
- **E.** The Student's t-test

QUESTION 83

The CVP trace

- **A.** The *c* wave follows the X descent
- **B.** The X descent occurs in (ventricular) diastole
- **C.** The *v* wave results from right atrial filling against a closed tricuspid valve
- **D.** Cannon waves are seen in complete heart block
- **E.** The *a* wave is of variable size in atrial fibrillation

QUESTION 84

Comparing methohexitone with thiopentone

A. Thiopentone has a higher pKa
B. Thiopentone is less ionized at pH 7.4
C. Thiopentone is more potent
D. Thiopentone is less protein bound
E. Thiopentone has a longer half life

QUESTION 85

Concerning failed rapid sequence induction

A. Prevention of aspiration is paramount
B. This was first considered in conjunction with obstetric intubation
C. Cricoid pressure should not be released
D. Transtracheal ventilation is the first manoeuvre to consider
E. The patient should be turned into the full left lateral

QUESTION 86

Spirometry is used for direct measurement of

A. Peak expiratory flow rate
B. Tidal volume
C. Vital capacity
D. Functional residual capacity
E. Expiratory reserve volume

QUESTION 87

Concerning coagulation and fibrinolysis

A. Thromboxane A2 inhibits platelet aggregation
B. Tissue thromboplastin activates factor VII
C. Antithrombin 3 is derived from activated factor X
D. Conversion of prothrombin to thrombin is calcium dependent
E. Factor XIII catalyses conversion of circulating fibrinogen to insoluble fibrin

QUESTION 88

Concerning 5–HT receptors

A. There are currently 3 major subdivisions
B. To date, the 5-HT$_1$ receptor has been divided into types A, B, and C
C. The anti-emetic ondansetron acts on 5-HT$_2$ receptors
D. They are found in the dorsal horn of the spinal cord
E. They can mediate both contraction and dilatation of the coronary vasculature

QUESTION 89

The following are features of theophylline toxicity

A. Theophylline has a narrow therapeutic index
B. Tremor
C. Petit mal type convulsions
D. Hyperkalaemia
E Rhabdomyolysis

QUESTION 90

Drugs with a high extraction ratio in the liver

A. Are likely to have low bioavailability if given orally
B. Will have an increased hepatic clearance following enzyme induction
C. Include etomidate
D. Include lignocaine
E. Require a high hepatic blood flow to be effectively cleared

Exam 2: Answers

ANSWER 1

A. FALSE   **B. FALSE**   **C. TRUE**   **D. TRUE**   **E. FALSE**

In man the essential amino acids are histidine, isoleucine, leucine, lysine, methionine, phenylalanine, threonine, tryptophan, and valine. 1 kCal = 4.2 kJ. The normal functional minimum protein intake is 1 g/kg/day. Essential fatty acids and the fat soluble vitamins (A,D,E,K) are required in the adult diet.

Ref: Despopoulos A, Silbernagl S. Color Atlas of Physiology. 196-231.

ANSWER 2

A. TRUE   **B. FALSE**   **C. FALSE**   **D. TRUE**   **E. FALSE**

At mains voltage (240 V) current flowing from one hand to the other across the trunk will show the following effects:

1-5 mA—tingling sensation

15-50 mA—skeletal muscle contraction ('no let go' leading to death from asphyxiation due to respiratory muscle paralysis

75-100 mA—ventricular fibrillation

>5 A—asystole or ventricular stand-still

Safety can be improved by isolating the patient from earth and so not completing the circuit. A residual current circuit breaker works by allowing current flow provided the neutral connector is at the same current as the live, so there is no leakage of current passing to earth. If the discrepancy in current flow at the neutral and live electrodes is greater than 30 mA the RCCB opens and the current flow is switched off.

Ref: Davey A, Moyle JTB, Ward CS. Ward's Anaesthetic Equipment, 3rd edn. W.B. Saunders, 1992

ANSWER 3

A. FALSE   **B. FALSE**   **C. FALSE**   **D. FALSE**   **E. FALSE**

The pattern of peripheral nerve stimulation used for assessment of neuromuscular blockade most commonly is the train-of-four. This shows characteristic fade when recovery from non-depolarising neuromuscular blockade is occurring. However in prolonged blockade with suxamethonium there is a conversion to the non-depolarising pattern with fade appearing. This is called dual block and occurs if the prolonged block is due to either repeated doses of suxamethonium or impaired metabolism (suxamethonium apnoea). The train-of-four is of no value when there is no response to the first twitch, and in this case post-tetanic count is used. During recovery it is difficult to assess the ratio between the first (T1) and fourth twitch (T4) and this should be 100:70 for successful extubation. This comparison is easier using the double burst pattern. Stimulators used for regional blockade should be used with the locating needle attached to the negative electrode as this ensures depolarisation of the nerve at a lower applied current.

Ref: Blunt MC, Urquhart JC. The Anaesthesia Viva: Physics, Measurement, Safety and Clinical Anaesthesia. Greenwich Medical Media, 1996

ANSWER 4

A. FALSE **B. TRUE** **C. FALSE** **D. TRUE** **E. FALSE**

Nitrous oxide is stored in cylinders painted blue overall in the UK (blue and white shoulders identify Entinox). The critical temperature of nitrous oxide is 36.5°C and therefore the cylinder contains liquid. It has a pressure equal to the saturated vapour pressure (approx. 52 bar at 20°C).

In order to measure the filling of a cylinder containing liquid it is impossible to use pressure (as this is constant at constant temperature) so filling ratio is used. This is equal to the mass of nitrous oxide divided by the mass of water that the cylinder can contain if full. The normal filling ratio in the UK is 0.67.

Ref: Blunt MC Urquhart JC. The Anaesthesia Viva: Physics, Measurement, Safety and Clinical Anaesthesia. Greenwich Medical Media., 1996

ANSWER 5

A. TRUE **B. TRUE** **C. FALSE** **D. FALSE** **E. FALSE**

Total lung capacity is equivalent to inspiratory capacity plus functional residual capacity (residual volume plus expiratory reserve volume). ATPS = Ambient temperature and pressure, saturated with water vapour.

Ref: Ganong WF. Review of Medical Physiology. Lange. Ch34.

ANSWER 6

A. FALSE **B. TRUE** **C. TRUE** **D. TRUE** **E. FALSE**

A and B fibres are myelinated and therefore have fast conduction velocities due to saltatory conduction. C fibres are unmyelinated. A-gamma fibres are motor to muscle spindles.

Ref: Ganong W F. Review of Medical Physiology. Lange.

ANSWER 7

A. FALSE **B. TRUE** **C. FALSE** **D. FALSE** **E. TRUE**

According to the alveolar gas equation:

$PAO_2 = (FiO_2 \times P_{atm}) - (PaCO_2 / RQ)$.

Hypoxic drive is negligible as long as PaO_2 remains above 8 kPa. As hypoxia develops, hyperventilation occurs, lowering $PaCO_2$ and allowing a higher PAO_2 for the same FiO_2. However, diminishing $PaCO_2$ reduces hypercarbic ventilatory drive and the two tend to balance one another at a maximum ventilatory rate x3 normal. Further rises in ventilatory rate must be made by conscious effort. Otherwise, unless supplementary oxygen is given or the ambient pressure is raised, unconsciousness ensues at PaO_2 <4.7 kPa. The normal subject breathing air at 3000 m has a PaO_2 of 8kPa. Below this altitude ventilation is controlled by hypercarbic drive. At 7000 m breathing air PaO_2 will be less than 4.7 kPa. At

10,000 m atmospheric pressure is 25 kPa. Normal PaO_2 can only be achieved by breathing supplementary oxygen or cabin pressurization. Acute altitude compensation occurs secondary to peripheral chemoreceptor stimulation by PaO_2 <8 kPa and leads to limited hyperventilation and tachycardia. Chronically, the ability to hyperventilate is extended by an increase in bicarbonate excretion which, by metabolic acidosis, compensates for the hyperventilation induced respiratory alkalosis. Oxygen delivery is further enhanced over time by an increased oxygen carrying capacity secondary to erythropoietin induced polycythaemia.

Ref: Despopoulos A, Silbernagl S. Color Atlas of Physiology, 108

ANSWER 8

A. FALSE   B. TRUE   C. FALSE   D. TRUE   E. TRUE

Ephedrine is a synthetic non-catecholamine which acts both directly and indirectly on alpha and beta adrenoreceptors. Cardiovascular effects last about ten times longer than adrenaline, but tachyphylaxis may be profound.

DOSE: 3-10 mg/kg increments iv (up to 50 mg)

ANSWER 9

A. TRUE   B. FALSE   C. FALSE   D. TRUE   E. FALSE

Heparin is a mucopolysaccharide acid present endogenously in the liver, mast cells and basophils. Onset time after IV injection is about 2 to 5 minutes. It is poorly lipid soluble and and has a high molecular weight and does not cross the placenta. It is metabolised by heparinase in the liver to inactive products.

Ref: Sasada, Smith. Drugs in Anaesthesia & Intensive Care

ANSWER 10

A. TRUE   B. TRUE   C. FALSE   D. FALSE   E. TRUE

In an over-resonant system the systolic will be over-estimated, the diastolic under-estimated and the mean accurate. In an over-damped system (eg due to air bubbles in the tubing) the systolic will be under-estimated, the diastolic over-estimated and the mean accurate. In an accurate trace, information can be obtained about the myocardial contractility and the systemic vascular resistance from the shape of the arterial waveform.

Ref: Yentis, Hirsch, Smith. Anaesthesia A to Z. Butterworth-Heinemann. Hutton, Cooper. Guidelines in Clinical Anaesthesia. Blackwell.

ANSWER 11

A. TRUE   B. TRUE   C. FALSE   D. FALSE   E. FALSE

The standard 2 litre adult reservoir bag is impregnated with carbon to make it antistatic. It can distend enormously holding 30 to 50 litres at least, however it will hold two litres without being forcibly distended. At maximum distension the pressure within the bag remains at about 40 to 50 cmH_2O until the bag fails. The bag may have a loop to allow it to be folded over (by hanging the loop from a hook on the top of the bag mount). This allows the movements of the bag to be more easily seen when anaesthetising children.

Ref: Davey A, Moyle JTB, Ward CS. Ward's Anaesthetic Equipment, 3rd edn. W.B. Saunders, 1992

ANSWER   12

A. FALSE   B. TRUE   C. FALSE   D. TRUE   E. TRUE

Venous return is reduced and therefore cardiac output; blood pressure is maintained by baroreceptor reflexes causing peripheral vasoconstriction; renin / angiotensin secretion is increased and cardiac output maintained by tachycardia in the face of a reduced stroke volume.

Ref: Ganong WF. Review of Medical Physiology. Lange. Ch31

ANSWER   13

A. TRUE   B. TRUE   C. FALSE   D. FALSE   E. TRUE

Cholestyramine interferes with the absorbtion of fat soluble vitamins thus potentiating the action of warfarin. Cimetidine potentiates the action by inhibiting the metabolism of the more potent S-form. Phenobarbitone and rifampicin induce the microsomal liver enzyme system enhancing the breakdown of anticoagulants. Tricyclics inhibit microsomal enzymes thus potentiating the effect.

ANSWER   14

A. TRUE   B. FALSE   C. FALSE   D. TRUE   E. FALSE

Clonidine and naphazoline have a higher affinity for alpha-2 receptors as does alpha-methylnoradrenaline, the metabolite of methyldopa, used for its action on central alpha-2 receptors to treat hypertension.

Ref: Maze, Tranquilli. Anesthesiology 1991; 74(3): 581

ANSWER   15

A. FALSE   B. TRUE   C. TRUE   D. FALSE   E. TRUE

$C/Co = e-kt$
C   = concentration at time t
Co = concentration at time zero
e   = 2.7183 the natural log base
k   = the rate constant

The rate constant k expresses the rate of concentration decline as a fraction of the concentration at that time. The time constant is 1/k and states the time taken for the concentration to decline to 36.8% (1/e) of its original value. The half life is the time taken for C to decline to half its initial value. Thus, at one half life C/Co=0.5

Therefore: ln 0.5 = -kt   =>   t = -(ln0.5 / k)   =>   t = 0.693 / k

Ref: Nunn, Utting, Brown. General Anaesthesia. Butterworths.

ANSWER   16

A. FALSE   B. TRUE   C. TRUE   D. TRUE   E. FALSE

The odds ratio is usually generated on a two-by-two table, with exposure on one axis and outcome on the other, and estimates the risk of the outcome given exposure to the postulated precipitant of that outcome. Statistical significance and clinical significance must not be confused.

ANSWER 17

A. FALSE   B. TRUE   C. TRUE   D. FALSE   E. FALSE

The null hypothesis sets out the assertion that a relationship between two samples does not exist; analytical statistical methods set about disproving the null hypothesis, in other words, demonstrating a relationship. The mode is the most commonly-observed value; the median is the measurement which lies exactly between each end of a range of values ranked in order.

ANSWER 18

A. FALSE   B. TRUE   C. FALSE   D. FALSE   E. TRUE

Hydroxyethyl starch is an amylopectin, a branched polysaccharide. The gelatins are produced from cattle bone and are urea linked or succinylated. Dextran 70 interferes with haemostasis in a dose dependent fashion. Haemaccel has a mean molecular weight of 35,000 (hydroxyethyl starch contains molecules with a weight average MW of 450,000 and a number average MW of 69,000). The half-life of hydroxyethyl starch is over 24 hours.

ANSWER 19

A. TRUE   B. TRUE   C. TRUE   D. FALSE   E. FALSE

Increased lithium levels are produced owing to an increase in lithium reabsorbtion. Amiodarone reduces the renal clearance of digoxin. Cimetidine inhibits cyt P_{450} leading to phenytoin toxicity. The interractions between beta blockers and verapamil, and ethanol and diazepam are pharmocodynamic.

ANSWER 20

A. TRUE   B. TRUE   C. FALSE   D. FALSE   E. FALSE

Flushing, hypertension and symptoms of ischaemic heart disease or cardiac failure may suggest this rare condition. Urinary elimination of metabolic products of catecholamines is diagnostic. Beta-blockade on its own must not be used without accompanying alpha-blockade, as systemic blood pressure may be elevated by unopposed alpha-adrenergic mediated vasoconstriction. Catecholamine levels do not revert to normal for 10 days and postoperative hypertensive crises are common - these patients should be managed on an intensive care unit with invasive monitoring for this reason. Steroid therapy is a feature of adrenal surgery and is not needed unless bilateral adrenalectomy is performed. Hypoglycaemia and hypotension due to hypovolaemia are also common in these patients.

ANSWER 21

A. FALSE   B. TRUE   C. FALSE   D. TRUE   E. TRUE

ACE Inhibitors are contraindicated in pregnancy, and in bilateral renal artery stenosis or unilateral renal artery stenosis supplying a single kidney as renal failure may supervene. They are probably best avoided in all cases of renovascular hypertension unless all other options have failed.

Ref: Anesthesia and Analgesia 1991: 72 (5): 667 BNF 1996

ANSWER 22

A. TRUE   B. FALSE   C. TRUE   D. TRUE   E. FALSE

Glomerular filtration is partly determined by molecular size, charge and protein binding. 99% glucose is reabsorbed by a saturable co-transport mechanism in the proximal tubule. Hydrogen ions are buffered intraluminally by phosphate.

Ref: Despopoulos A, Silbernagl S. Color Atlas of Physiology. 120-150.

ANSWER 23

A. FALSE   B. FALSE   C. FALSE   D. TRUE   E. TRUE

The Clark or polarographic electrode is used to measure oxygen concentration in blood. It consists of a silver/silver chloride anode, a platinum cathode and an electrolyte medium which is allowed to reach equilibrium with the sample. This medium is normally either potassium chloride or hydroxide. The electrodes are connected by a battery and when a voltage of 0.6 V is applied across them a current flows proportional to the amount of oxygen in the electrolyte medium. The reaction at the cathode is similar to that seen in the mitochondrion: $O2 + 4e^- + 2H_2O \rightarrow 4(OH)^-$

Ref: Davis PD, Parbrook GD, Kenny GNC. Basic Physics and Measurement in Anaesthesia, 4th edn. Butterworth-Heinemann, 1995

ANSWER 24

A. FALSE   B. FALSE   C. TRUE   D. TRUE   E. FALSE

SA and AV action potentials do not have a plateau phase. The action potential begins with a maximum diastolic potential of about -70 mV which slowly depolarizes until a threshold potential of about -40 mV when rapid depolarization occurs (calcium and potassium conductance rise). Vagal stimulation results in an increased K conductance that flattens the prepotential slope and increases the negativity of the maximum diastolic potential. Sympathetic stimulation causes an increase in Ca conductance that increases the slope of the prepotential allowing the threshold potential to be attained more rapidly. Hypothermia flattens the prepotential gradient giving rise to a negative chronotropic effect.

Ref: Despopoulos A, Silbernagl S. Color Atlas of Physiology, 154-191

ANSWER 25

A. FALSE   B. FALSE   C. TRUE   D. TRUE   E. FALSE

Ondansetron is a highly selective and competive 5-HT antagonist acting at the third receptor subtype which can be given intravenously or orally. It has a half life of 3 hours. It undergoes extensive hepatic metabolism by hydroxylation and glucoronide conjugation. The most common side effects are constipation and mild headache. It has not been associated with sedation or extrapyramidal effects.

Ref: Nimmo, Smith: Anaesthesia: chapter 19

ANSWER 26

A. FALSE   B. TRUE   C. TRUE   D. TRUE   E. TRUE

The trans-trans isomer makes up 54-64%, the cis-trans isomer 32-38%, and the cis-cis isomer 4-8%. In patients with end-stage liver disease, the duration of action of mivacurium is prolonged up to three-fold, primarily due to decreased plasma cholinesterase activity. Most of the unwanted effects of mivacurium can be ascribed to the release of histamine.

ANSWER   27

A. TRUE   B. FALSE   C. FALSE   D. TRUE   E. FALSE

CO_2 (unlike H^+ & HCO_3^-) rapidly diffuses across the blood-brain barrier, enabling the PCO_2 of CSF to adjust quickly to changes in PCO_2 of blood. In the absence of blood cells and non-bicarbonate buffers, pH changes in the CSF are more marked, and these are registered by central chemoreceptors. Slow equilibration of HCO_3 allows chronic adaptation. The blood solubility coefficient of $CO_2 = 0.0225$ mmol/l/kPAa or 0.03 mmol/l/mmHg. Transport of CO_2 on Hb is reduced in the presence of HbO_2 by the Haldane effect. CO_2 gives rise to increased activation of the sympathetic system.

Ref: Ganong WF. Review of Medical Physiology, Lange

ANSWER   28

A. TRUE   B. FALSE   C. FALSE   D. FALSE   E. FALSE

Absolute refractory period = 1-3 ms, the action potential lasts 2-4 ms. Thin filaments originating at the Z-line are made up from actin and tropomyosin chains with troponin molecules located at intervals. Myosin chains are thick and form A-bands of constant width. The thin filaments slide in between the myosin filaments and cross linkages form between actin & myosin. Contraction is initiated by binding of calcium to troponin-C. Calmodulin binds calcium in smooth muscle.

Ref: Ganong WF. Review of Medical Physiology. Lange, Ch3

ANSWER   29

A. FALSE   B. TRUE   C. FALSE   D. TRUE   E. TRUE

Iron is absorbed to replace losses (normally greater in women and 3-6% of ingested iron). Ferrous form is more readily absorbed and this is formed by reduction of ferric iron in the stomach. Vitamin C in the diet also facilitates reduction. Absorption occurs mainly in the upper small intestine.

Ref: Ganong WF. Review of Medical Physiology. Lange, Ch25

ANSWER   30

A. TRUE   B. TRUE   C. TRUE   D. FALSE   E. FALSE

Thiazides tend to result in hypokalaemic, hypochloraemic metabolic alkalosis. Thiazide diuretics can cause hypercalcaemia and hyperglycaemia.

ANSWER   31

A. FALSE   B. TRUE   C. TRUE   D. FALSE   E. TRUE

Flow through tubes may be either ordered (laminar) or disordered (turbulent). As the flow velocity increases a point is reached above which flow tends to be turbulent (this is the critical velocity). Thus a fast-flowing river is disrupted and turbulent whilst the slow stream is smooth and laminar. This was described in smooth-sided tubes by Reynolds and his formula shows an increase as the velocity increases. Reynolds number = (mean velocity x density x diameter)/ viscosity). However turbulence will also occur locally if the flow is disrupted by the characteristics of flowpath (water flowing round a rock in a stream will show turbulent eddies downstream). An example of this is the angled connector normally used for endotracheal tubes. Laminar flow has a parabolic pattern with flow in the centre being faster and that at the peripheries almost stationary.Helium is used in anaesthesia because it has a low density. This makes its flow much higher in turbulent conditions such as in upper airway obstruction .(e.g. epiglottitis). Helium flow in laminar conditions is similar to oxygen.

Ref: Mushin WM, Jones PL. Physics for the Anaesthetist, 4th edn. Blackwell Scientific Publications, 1987

ANSWER 32

A. TRUE   B. FALSE   C. TRUE   D. FALSE   E. FALSE

T4 & T3 are synthesized in the colloid by iodination and condensation of tyrosine molecules and bound in thyroglobulin. Colloid is ingested during secretion and T4 & T3 released from thyroglobulin. Peipheral conversion of T4 to T3 can occur by deiodination.

Ref: Ganong WF. Review of Medical Physiology. Lange. Ch18.

ANSWER 33

A. TRUE   B. FALSE   C. TRUE   D. FALSE   E. TRUE

Glucagon is formed in the pancreatic A-cells. Secretion is stimulated by B-mediated sympathetic nerves to the pancreas, amino acids, CCK, gastrin, cortisol, infection, Ach, and theophylline; but inhibited by alpha stimulation, insulin, glucose, ketones, phenytoin and somatostatin. Glucagon is gluconeogenic, glycogenolytic, and lipolytic.

Ref: Ganong WF. Review of Medical Physiology. Lange, Ch19

ANSWER 34

A. TRUE   B. TRUE   C. TRUE   D. TRUE   E. FALSE

Gentamicin is poorly lipid soluble and therefore is given parenterally. It undergoes extensive renal excretion due exclusively to glomerular filtration. About 60% is excreted unchanged in the first 24 hours. Aminoglycosides tend to potentiate neuromuscular blockade by inhibition of presynaptic acetyl choline release and by stabilisation of the post synaptic membrane at the neuromuscular junction.

Ref: Sasada, Smith. Drugs in Anaesthesia and Intensive Care.

ANSWER 35

A. TRUE   B. FALSE   C. FALSE   D. TRUE   E. TRUE

It is less than 50% protein bound. It does not contain a sulphydryl group and therefore cannot be expected to scavenge free radicals.

Ref: Anaesthesia 1994; 49(7): 613

ANSWER 36

A. TRUE   B. TRUE   C. FALSE   D. FALSE   E. FALSE

PTH is released in response to hypocalcaemia. It acts on the intestine indirectly by stimulating the conversion of 25-OH cholecalciferol to 1,25-diOH cholecalciferol in the kidneys. This D-hormone (a steroid) mineralizes bone and enhances gut calcium absorption. PTH also stimulates osteoclasts and inhibits phosphate reabsorption in the kidneys whilst increasing calcium reabsorption.

Ref: Despopoulos A, Silbernagl S. Color Atlas of Physiology, 232-271

ANSWER 37

A.FALSE   **B. FALSE**   **C. FALSE**   **D. TRUE**   **E. FALSE**

Nifedipine is a dihyropyridine derivative. Verapamil is a papaverine derivative. Nifedipine is absorbed more rapidly (2 min) after intranasal administration compared to sublingual (3-5 min). Unlike verapamil, it does not undergo significant first pass metabolism, and is metabolised wholly to inert products. There are three inactive metabolites.

Ref: Sasada, Smith. Drugs in Anaesthesia & Intensive Care

ANSWER 38

A. TRUE   **B. TRUE**   **C. FALSE**   **D. FALSE**   **E. FALSE**

Neostigmine and suxamethonium can cause prolonged contraction which may be impossible to reverse. Suxamethonium can also cause extreme potassium release. The condition is exacerbated by cold, but may be precipitated by muscular activity (percussion myotonia). Testicular atrophy and endocrine insufficiency are also associations. Procyclidine is used to treat the dystonic reactions seen with major tranquillizers and metoclopramide. It has no place in the management of this condition. These patients are at risk of cardiac dysrhythmias and aspiration due to poor bulbar function. Respiratory function is very sensitive to both opiates and muscle relaxants.

Ref: Russell et al. Anaesthesia and myotonia. British Journal of Anaesthesia 1994;72:210.

ANSWER 39

A. TRUE   **B. FALSE**   **C. FALSE**   **D. TRUE**   **E. TRUE**

Cocaine paste is opaque and obscures the view; phenylephrine is preferred. The nasal route is technically easier but many prefer the oral route. The technique is used for unstable neck fractures, known or anticipated difficult intubations, and also for endobronchial tubes where accurate placement can be confirmed.

ANSWER 40

A. FALSE   **B. TRUE**   **C. TRUE**   **D. FALSE**   **E. TRUE**

Pancreatic juice is alkaline, rich in bicarbonate and secreted under both humoral and vagal control.

Ref: Ganong WF. Review of Medical Physiology, Lange

ANSWER 41

A. TRUE   **B. TRUE**   **C. FALSE**   **D. FALSE**   **E. FALSE**

Blood flow (ml /100 g/min) to various organs: Liver = 57, kidneys = 420, Brain = 54, Skin = 13, Sk. muscle = 2.7, Heart = 84.

Ref: Ganong WF. Review of Medical Physiology. Lange. Ch32.

ANSWER 42

A. FALSE   B. TRUE   C. TRUE   D. FALSE   E. TRUE

Acute porphyric attacks are induced by alcohol, diet, pregnancy and in the case of the hepatic forms of the condition by barbiturates and steroids. Induction of d-aminolaevulinic acid synthetase with a deficiency of an enzyme further down the pathway of haem synthesis underlies all forms. Tourniquets, hypoxia and acidosis induce sickle crises not porphyria. Safe anaesthesia includes propofol, vecuronium, opiates and domperidone. Volatiles are probably not safe, and the use of local anaesthetic agents is contentious.

Ref: Harrison et al. Anaesthesia for the porphyric patient. Anaesthesia 1993;48:417

ANSWER 43

A. FALSE   B. FALSE   C. TRUE   D. TRUE   E. FALSE

The correlation coefficient is denoted by the symbol "r". It varies from -1 to +1 and is normally represented by the gradient of a best fit line applied to a scatter plot of the two variables in question. Complete correlation of the two variables is expressed by 1. The +ve or -ve sign denote the relationship (increasing or decreasing) between the two variables. Linked variables will always have a degree of correlation.

Ref: Swinscow. Statistics at Square One. BMJ Publications

ANSWER 44

A. TRUE   B. FALSE   C. TRUE   D. FALSE   E. FALSE

Edrophonium is about ten times less potent than neostigmine. About 75% is eliminated via the kidney. It is poorly lipid soluble and is not therefore given orally. Unlike neostigmine, it does not inhibit plasma cholinesterase. Its trade name is "Tensilon" and it is used in the diagnosis of myasthenia gravis.

ANSWER 45

A. TRUE   B. TRUE   C. TRUE   D. TRUE   E. FALSE

Pain occurs in up to 80% of patients, and myoclonic movements in about 30%. PONV is common and the incidence is higher than with other agents. It is hydrolysed in the liver and the metabolites excreted in the urine. The main metabolites are not active. It is metabolised by plasma esterases but this does not appear to occur in humans. It is formulated in 35% propylene glycol with a pH of 4.1.

PHYSICAL:
    pH 4.1, 75% protein bound
DOSE:
    0.2-0.3 mg/kg iv

Ref: Nimmo, Rowbotham, Smith. Anaesthesia. Blackwell, Chapter 6

ANSWER 46

A. TRUE   B. TRUE   C. FALSE   D. TRUE   E. TRUE

This rare syndrome is characterised by extra-pyramidal signs, deterioration in mental status, autonomic lability and hyperthermia. It is precipitated by phenothiazines and butyrephenones. It has similar features to malignant hyperpyrexia from which it may be indistinguishable in the anaesthetised patient.

ANSWER 47

A. TRUE   B. FALSE   C. TRUE   D. FALSE   E. FALSE

Pressure within the pleural cavity can be measured indirectly using an oesophageal balloon. In spontaneous respiration it is negative (due to the thoracic cage's tendency to spring outwards and the lungs' tendency to collapse inwards). It increases in magnitude as lung volume increases (thus becomes more negative during inspiration) and in the erect posture it is more negative (lower) at the apex of the lung than at the bases. It will become positive during IPPV. The total partial pressures of gases dissolved in blood (and therefore tissues) is always less than atmospheric so the pleural cavity is kept free from gas.

Ref: Nunn JF. Applied Respiratory Physiology. Butterworth-Heinemann

ANSWER 48

A. TRUE   B. TRUE   C. TRUE   D. FALSE   E. TRUE

Ref: Seminars in Anesthesia 1995; 14(1): 46

ANSWER 49

A. FALSE   B. TRUE   C. TRUE   D. TRUE   E. FALSE

CEMD has been reporting every three years since 1952 and since 1985 has included Scotland. The biggest killers continue to be hypertensive disease and pulmonary embolism.

Ref: NCEPOD

ANSWER 50

A. FALSE   B. TRUE   C. FALSE   D. FALSE   E. TRUE

It is a fluorinated 4-quinolone. It has a wide spectrum of activity against Gram negative organisms but its activity against Gram positive organisms is questionable. It is well absorbed when taken by mouth, with good bioavailability.

ANSWER 51

A. FALSE   B. FALSE   C. FALSE   D. TRUE   E. FALSE

Desflurane is a fluorinated methyl ethyl ether. It has a boiling pont of 23.5 degrees C compared to 48.5 degrees C for isoflurane and so requires special vapouriser technology for delivery into a standard anaesthetic circuit. Isoflurane and enflurane have the same molecular weight (184.5) as they are structural isomers. The molecular weight of desflurane being 168 with a MAC of about 6%. About 0.02% is metabolised (the least metabolised of the commonly used volatile agents). It has the same basic structure as isoflurane and enflurane but is the fluorinated derivative with greater stablility. Remember halothane is a hydrocarbon and sevoflurane a methyl propyl ether.

Ref: Graham. The desflurane TEC 6 vaporizer. British Journal of Anaesthesia 1994; 72: 470-473

ANSWER 52

A. TRUE   B. FALSE   C. FALSE   D. FALSE   E. FALSE

It is composed of two molecules of acetylcholine, but is metabolised to the relatively inactive succinyl monocholine. The rise in intraocular pressure caused by suxamethonium alone is brief, lasting for a few minutes. The bradycardia is caused by activation of muscarinic receptors. Phase II block does exhibit the characteristics of non-depolarising block but is not reversed by anticholinesterases.

ANSWER 53

A. TRUE   B. TRUE   C. TRUE   D. TRUE   E. TRUE

Under basal conditions carbohydrate = 35%, ketones & amino acids = 5%, fat = 60%. Circulating free fatty acids account for 50% of lipid utilized. Anaerobic metabolism acounts for less than 1%.

Ref: Ganong WF. Review of Medical Physiology. Lange, Ch3

ANSWER 54

A. FALSE   B. FALSE   C. FALSE   D. TRUE   E. TRUE

Aortic pressure is highest in mid-systole. Left atrial pressure is highest in early diastole. Aortic blood flow is lowest in early diastole. Aortic pressure exceeds left ventricular pressure late in systole for a short time but momentum keeps the blood flowing. A fourth heart sound is due to filling of a stiff ventricle and is heard during atrial systole.

Ref: Ganong WF. Review of Medical Physiology. Lange.

ANSWER 55

A. TRUE   B. TRUE   C. FALSE   D. FALSE   E. FALSE

Basophils are not phagocytic, eosinophils attack parasites whereas neutrophils defend against bacteria. T lymphocytes originate in the thymus gland.

Ref: Ganong WF. Review of Medical Physiology. Lange. Ch27.

ANSWER 56

A. TRUE   B. TRUE   C. FALSE   D. FALSE   E. TRUE

Potassium = 160:5, Magnesium = 28:2, Chloride = 3:110, Bicarbonate = 10:27, Phosphate = 100:2.

Ref: Despopoulos A, Silbernagl S. Color Atlas of Physiology. 60-77

ANSWER 57

A. FALSE   B. FALSE   C. TRUE   D. FALSE   E. TRUE

The Mallampati system detects only 50% of difficult intubations. Grade 1 allows a full view down to the tip of the uvula, grade 2 the base of the uvula, grade 3 the soft palate only and grade 4 is where the soft palate cannot be seen. The Wilson test is of ability to protrude the mandible below the maxilla, where A is the mandible beyond the maxilla, B is where they can be aligned, and C is where the mandible cannot be brought in line with the maxilla. Neck extension is more important than flexion, and may reveal vertebro-basilar insufficiency in the susceptible.

Ref: Recognition and management of difficult airway problems. Cobley M, Vaughan R. British Journal of Anaesthesia 1992;68:90-97.

ANSWER 58

A. TRUE   B. FALSE   C. TRUE   D. FALSE   E. TRUE

Respiratory nitrogen measurement is performed by either Raman scattering or mass spectrometry. It is valuable to ensure the adequacy of denitrogenation during pre-oxygenation. In the early stages of general anaesthesia a rapid fall in respiratory nitrogen is expected. If this fails to happen there may be a leak in the circuit. Nitrogen analysis has been recommended for use during neurosurgery as a way to differentiate air embolus from other events causing a fall in end-tidal carbon dioxide.

Ref: Dorsch JA, Dorsch SE. Understanding Anesthesia Equipment; Construction, Care and Complications, 2nd edn. Williams & Wilkins, 1984

ANSWER 59

A. TRUE   B. TRUE   C. FALSE   D. TRUE   E. FALSE

First described for the assessment of head injury, it is now used for all types of coma. It is most usefully broken down into the components of

best motor response (1-6)

best verbal response (1-5)

eye opening (1-4)

change over time is a more useful guide to progress than is a single measurement. A score of 2 is not possible as 3 is the lowest score.

ANSWER 60

A. FALSE   B. TRUE   C. TRUE   D. FALSE   E. TRUE

ANSWER 61

A.TRUE   B.TRUE   C.TRUE   D. FALSE   E. TRUE

Pulse oximetry relies on measuring the relative absorbance at two wavelengths (660nm and 940nm). Reduced haemoglobin has greater absorbance at 660nm and oxyhaemoglobin greater at 940nm. The ratio is the determined and the SpO_2 is then calculated. The monitor is accurate to within 3% at values of over 70%, but less accurate as the saturation falls. Other molecules in the blood may affect the value of SpO_2. Carboxyhaemoglobin causes an increase in SpO_2 equal to its concentration, but methaemoglobin absorbs light equally at both 660nm and 940nm so the saturation tends towards a value of 85%. Fetal haemoglobin does not however affect the accuracy of pulse oximetry.

Ref: Tremper KK, Wahr JA. Advances in respiratory monitoring. In: Sanford TJ (Ed) Clinical Issues in Monitoring. W.B. Saunders, 1994, pp 261-276

ANSWER 62

A. TRUE   B. FALSE   C. TRUE   D. FALSE   E. FALSE

There are many afferent inputs to the vomiting centre and the limbic system is one (hence 'nauseating smells' and 'sickening sights'.) The vomiting centre is situated in the area postrema in the lateral walls of the 4th ventricle. During vomiting the glottis closes and the breath is held in mid-inspiration.

Ref: Ganong WF. Review of Medical Physiology. Lange

ANSWER 63

A. FALSE   B. FALSE   C. FALSE   D. TRUE   E. TRUE

Surgical diathermy relies on the heating effect of an electrical current. It has a very high frequency (>100 kHz) and this avoids the danger of excitation of skeletal or cardiac muscle.

Unipolar diathermy relies on the passage from the active electrode (which is small and so has a high current density) to a distant 'plate' electrode which is coupled to ground by a capacitor. The current passes to the earth via the route of least resistance. If the resistance of the plate electrode is large then the current may be able to pass to earth via another route, such as the ECG electrodes. As these are small there is a larger current density at this point and so burning can occur.

Bipolar diathermy relies on the passage of current between two electrodes close together. This minimises the passage of current through the body and so avoids the risk of problems with pacemakers.

It should be remembered that flammable anaesthetic agents are not the only combustible gases in theatre, and fires have been reported from surgical cleaning agents as well as explosions from gas within the bowel.

Ref: Sykes MK, Vickers MD, Hull CJ. Principles of Measurement and Monitoring in Anaesthesia and Intensive Care, 3rd edn. Blackwell Scientific Publishers, 1991

ANSWER 64

A. FALSE   B. FALSE   C. FALSE   D. FALSE   E. FALSE

An oxygen failure warning device must be fitted to all anaesthetic machines. According to British Standard (BS 4272 Pt 3) the device must be auditory and last for at least 7 seconds at a volume of 60 dB. It must be solely powered by the oxygen supply pressure. It must be designed so it CANNOT be switched off before the oxygen supply is reconnected. The alarm should activate as the pressure falls below 200kPa and the gas supply should be either progressively reduced as the oxygen fails or replaced with oxygen or air.

Ref: Davey A, Moyle JTB, Ward CS. Ward's Anaesthetic Equipment, 3rd edn. W.B. Saunders, 1992

ANSWER 65

A. TRUE   B. FALSE   C. TRUE   D. TRUE   E. TRUE

Lipid soluble agents are transfered across the placenta. Weak acids and bases are transferred in their non-ionised form. Polarised molecules such as neuromuscular blockers are not transferred at all.

Ref: Urquhart J, Blunt M. The Anaesthesia Viva: volume 1.

ANSWER 66

A. FALSE   B. FALSE   C. TRUE   D. TRUE   E. FALSE

Optic nerve lesions cause unilateral loss of vision. Optic chiasm lesions cause bitemporal hemianopia since it is here that the temporal fibres cross the midline. Optic tract lesions cause homonymous hemianopia since the optic tracts carry fibres that supply the same field (ie left or right) from both eyes. Lesions of the geniculocalcarine tract and the occipital cortex often spare the macula because the macula fibres are separated from the rest of the cortex subserving vision.

Ref: Ganong WF. Review of Medical Physiology. Lange.

ANSWER   67

A. TRUE   B. TRUE   C. TRUE   D. TRUE   E. FALSE

All the volatile agents enhance the action of neuromuscular blockers by reducing the tone of skeletal muscle, an action mediated by an effect at the post junctional membrane. Quinidine is a membrane stabiliser and an isomer of quinine. Dantrolene disrupts excitation-contraction coupling and so does not directly potentiate the action of NMBs.

Ref: Sasada, Smith. Drugs in Anaesthesia and Intensive Care.

ANSWER   68

A. TRUE   B. TRUE   C. FALSE   D. FALSE   E. TRUE

CSF is secreted by the choroid plexuses in the IIIrd, IVth and lateral ventricles. It passes through the foramina of Monro to reach the IIIrd ventricle from the lateral ventricles, and leaves the IVth ventricle via the foramina of Magendie and Luschka. It passes into the dural venous sinuses via the arachnoid villi. Its formation is due to secretion and filtration of plasma and is largely independant of ICP, but removal increases with increasing pressure.

Ref: Yentis, Hirsch, Smith. Anaesthesia A to Z. Butterworth-Heinemann

ANSWER   69

A. FALSE   B. TRUE   C. FALSE   D. TRUE   E. FALSE

The electrocardiogram was the first commonly available monitor in theatre use. It measures current flowing in the heart in various directions. If there is no current flow then the ECG is 'zero'. However between complexes the heart is normally at a common resting potential of approximately -50 to -70 mV but as there is no current flowing the ECG is 'zero'. Electrical activity in the heart starts with depolarisation that flows from the SA node to the AV node via the atria and then down the Purkinje fibres and outward to the muscle tissue. The repolarisation that then occurs progresses in the opposite direction (thus the T wave is upright). In order to ascertain both rhythm and ischaemic information leads II and V_5 are recommended, but a modification of lead V_5 (CM_5) has been developed in an attempt to get this information from one ECG channel. ECG electrodes are silver/silver chloride electrodes.

ANSWER   70

A. FALSE   B. TRUE   C. TRUE   D. FALSE   E. FALSE

Ropivacaine is a pure enantiomer, existing as the S(-) isomer. This has been found to be less toxic and more potent than the R-isomer. It is more effective than equipotent doses of bupivacaine at blocking Ad and C fibres while being about 15% less depressant on motor fibres. It is half as lipid soluble as bupivacaine. Its clearance is 30% greater than bupivacaine. In addition the dose required to produce toxicity is consistently 1.5-2 times that of bupivacaine.

Ref: Seminars in Anesthesia March 1996

ANSWER   71

A. TRUE   B. FALSE   C. FALSE   D. TRUE   E. FALSE

Dantrolene will potentiate the action of the NDMRs but this is rarely of clinical significance. It has been used in the treatment of the neuroleptic malignant syndrome as has bromocriptine but neither are reliable treatments.

Ref: BNF 1996

ANSWER 72

A. TRUE   B. TRUE   C. TRUE   D. FALSE   E. FALSE

Soda lime consists of:
Calcium hydroxide (approx. 75-80%)
Potassium hydroxide (1%)
Sodium hydroxide (4%)
Water (14-19%)
Silica and kieselguhr as hardeners
Indicator dye

Ref: Dorsch JA, Dorsch SE.Understanding Anesthesia Equipment; Construction, Care and Complications, 2nd edn. Williams & Wilkins, 1984

ANSWER 73

A. FALSE   B. TRUE   C. FALSE   D. TRUE   E. FALSE

The dermatomal level of analgesia is important to record for continuation of adequate post-operative analgesia, and in order to ensure that a patient is not returned to the ward with a dangerously-high level of block. The requirement is for one nurse per patient. Oxygen is recommended for transfer of immediately-postoperative patients. NSAID are contraindicated in bronchospasm, peptic ulceration, dehydration and renal impairment. Oliguria must never be treated with a diuretic without knowledge of the state of hydration; the first line is a fluid challenge.

Ref: Association of Anaesthetists

ANSWER 74

A. FALSE   B. FALSE   C. TRUE   D. TRUE   E. FALSE

Cardiac output increases by 40%, due to an increase in heart rate and a 30% increase in stroke volume. Both SVR and mean arterial blood pressure fall.

Ref: Yentis, Hirsch, Smith. Anaesthesia A to Z. Butterworth-Heinemann.

ANSWER 75

A. TRUE   B. FALSE   C. TRUE   D. TRUE   E. TRUE

In sickle cell disease the beta globin chains are abnormal (although rate of synthesis is normal, c.f. thalassaemias) due to a mutation of adenine to thymine causing a substitution of glutamic acid for valine in the amino acid chain. This causes red cells to sickle ie form crystals at low oxygen tensions thus leading to vascular infarcts. Its distribution parallels that of pl. falciparum malaria against which it confers some protection. It is generally more severe in Africans.

Ref: Nimmo, Rowbotham, Smith. Anaesthesia. Blackwell.

ANSWER 76

A. FALSE   B. TRUE   C. FALSE   D. TRUE   E. FALSE

In the neonate, the right main bronchus lies at the same angle to the trachea as the left main bronchus, so inadvertent endobronchial intubation is less likely. Valveless breathing systems do offer an advantage, but because of reduction in resistance, entrainment of room air occurs if the limb of the breathing system is less than tidal volume, not minute volume. The fresh gas flow must exceed 3 l/minute for the same reason. Tracheal tube size is calculated popularly by size in mm = age/4 + 4.

Ref: Davey A, Moyle JTB, Ward CS. Ward's Anaesthetic Equipment, 3rd edn. WB Saunders, 1992

ANSWER 77

A. TRUE B. FALSE C. TRUE D. FALSE E. TRUE

Only pacemaker tissue has pre-potentials and demonstrates rhythmic discharge. The pre-potentials of pacemaker tissue are due to potassium ions and the SA node has the shortest pre-potential.

Ref: Ganong WF. Review of Medical Physiology. Lange.

ANSWER 78

A. TRUE B. TRUE C. FALSE D. TRUE E. TRUE

A kcal = 1000 cal or 4.185 kJ. In the body, fats and carbohydrates are completely oxidized to CO_2 and H_2O so that the available and physical calorific values are identical. Proteins are incompletely oxidized to CO_2: they form urea etc. as end products. Therefore the available calorific value (4.1 kcal/g) is less than the physical calorific value (5.7 kcal/g) that would be obtained by complete combustion to H_2O, CO_2 etc. in a bomb calorimeter. The metabolic rate rises with a protein diet because 89kJ are required to produce 1 mol ATP from amino acids, but only 74 kJ if the source is carbohydrate.

Ref: Despopoulos A, Silbernagl S. Color Atlas of Physiology, 196-231

ANSWER 79

A. FALSE B. TRUE C. FALSE D. TRUE E. FALSE

Oxygen must be administered and airway obstruction must be excluded. Naloxone should not be given blindly. The effects of a single dose of suxamethonium cannot be reversed by neostigmine. Indeed it may worsen the situation and enhance phase II block. A nerve stimulator, correctly applied, may identify incomplete reversal of neuromuscular blockade as the cause. This may be either prolonged suxamethonium action, phase II block or prolonged non-depolarising block. Carbon dioxide is best reserved for putting out fires! Hypokalaemia, hypermagnesaemia, hypocalcaemia and hypothermia all enhance the effects of neuromuscular block.

ANSWER 80

A. FALSE B. FALSE C. TRUE D. FALSE E. TRUE

Depth of anaesthesia is very difficult to monitor. The risk of inadequate anaesthesia when the patient is paralysed and unable to communicate (known as 'awareness') is one of the main stimuli behind the attempt to find a reliable, repeatable monitor of depth of anaesthesia. This problem came to light in the 1950's when oxygen/nitrous oxide anaesthesia was commonly used with muscle relaxation. The addition of opioids, even in high dose did not abolish the problem. The incidence of awareness in obstetric anaesthesia is now variously quoted between 0.4 % and 7 %. The incidence in general surgery is still significant but lower (0.1 to 1%). Attempts to monitor depth of anaesthesia have included the use of the EEG and modifications of it and of lower oesophageal contractility measurement (the contractility decreasing in amplitude and frequency with increasing depth of anaesthesia).

These have not proved to be reliable. Other methods tried include the isolated-arm technique and evoked potentials. At present medium latency (early cortical) auditory evoked potentials seem to be the technique showing most promise.

Ref: Faust RJ (ed). Anesthesiology Review, 2nd edn. Churchill Livingstone, 1994

ANSWER 81

A. FALSE   B. TRUE   C. FALSE   D. TRUE   E. TRUE

The motor cortex is made up of pyramidal cells in the pre-central gyrus region (the post-central region is somatosensory). Legs are represented uppermost and regions that require fine motor control (eg hands) have a disproportionately large representation. Most fibres decussate in the lower medulla and then continue as lateral corticospinal tracts, however some fibres pass uncrossed in the anterior corticospinal tract then cross within the spinal cord at their spinal level.

Ref: Yentis, Hirsch, Smith. Anaesthesia A to Z. Butterworth-Heinemann.

ANSWER 82

A. TRUE   B. TRUE   C. TRUE   D. FALSE   E. FALSE

Non-parametric tests are applied to data that is not normally distributed, or to data where the distribution is not known. The commonly used non-parametric tests are the Mann-Whitney (for ordinal data), and the Chi-squared (for nominal data). The Wilcoxon signed rank sum test is used to compare two groups and the same subjects before and after a treatment.

Ref: Yentis, Hirsch, Smith. Anaesthesia A to Z. Butterworth-Heinemann

ANSWER 83

A. FALSE   B. FALSE   C. TRUE   D. TRUE   E. FALSE

The CVP trace consists of three main waves and two descents, (in chronological order):

The a wave - right atrial (RA) contraction. Absent in atrial fibrillation; enlarged with tricuspid stenosis, RV hypertrophy, pulmonary stenosis or pulmonary hypertension; cannon waves (giant A waves) occur if the RA contracts against a closed tricuspid valve (e.g. in complete heart block)

The c wave - bulging of the tricuspid valve at the onset of ventricular systole

The X descent - atrial relaxation during ventricular systole

The v wave - RA filling with a closed tricuspid valve

The Y descent - opening of the tricuspid valve with blood flow into the right ventricle.

Ref: Faust RJ (ed) Anesthesiology Review, 2nd edn. Churchill Livingstone, 1994

ANSWER 84

A. FALSE   B. FALSE   C. FALSE   D. FALSE   E. TRUE

THIOPENTONE
    Dose = 5mg/kg
    pKa = 7.6
    Protein binding = 85%
    Unionized fraction at pH 7.4 = 61%

Initial T 1/2 = 8.5 mins

Terminal T 1/2 = 11.6 hrs

METHOHEXITONE

Dose = 1mg/kg

pKa = 7.9

Protein binding = 85%

Unionized fraction at pH 7.4 = 75%

Initial T 1/2 = 5.6 mins

Terminal T 1/2 = 3.9 hrs

Ref: Nunn, Utting, Brown. General Anaesthesia. Butterworths.

ANSWER 85

A. FALSE   **B. TRUE**   **C. TRUE**   **D. FALSE**   **E. TRUE**

Oxygenation is the first priority of any of the published variations of the failed intubation drill, the earliest of which was described by Mike Tunstall in Aberdeen in connection with obstetrics. Full left lateral, continuation of oxygenation with cricoid pressure and obtaining assistance are the priorities. Many would now advocate use of the laryngeal mask with continuation of cricoid pressure. Transtracheal ventilation is a last resort.

ANSWER 86

A. FALSE   **B. TRUE**   **C. TRUE**   **D. FALSE**   **E. TRUE**

Spirometry allows measurement of lung volumes by recording expiratory and inspiratory volumes. It is not used to measure expiratory flow rate and because it cannot measure residual lung volume it cannot measure FRC directly. It can measure all other lung volumes (including expiratory reserve volume, tidal volume and vital capacity).

Ref: Urquhart JC,   Blunt MC. The Anaesthesia Viva: Physiology, Pharmacology and Statistics, Greenwich Medical Media, 1996

ANSWER 87

A. FALSE   **B. TRUE**   **C. TRUE**   **D. TRUE**   **E. FALSE**

Thromboxane A2 promotes platelet aggregation but is opposed by simultaneous formation of prostacyclin (PGI2). Activation of the extrinsic pathway by tissue thromboplastin involves factor VII. Fibrinogen is converted to loose fibrin by thrombin and is further converted to a tight aggregate by the catalytic action of factor XIII.

Ref: Ganong WF. Review of Medical Physiology. Lange, Ch27

ANSWER 88

A. FALSE   **B. FALSE**   **C. FALSE**   **D. TRUE**   **E. TRUE**

5-HT (serotonin) is synthesised from the amino acid precursor tryptophan derived from the diet. It is found in intestine, CNS and platelets (not neutrophils). It is metabolised by enzymes located in many tissues, including liver and brain. The measurement of urinary 5-HIAA is utilised in the diagnosis of carcinoid syndrome.There are currently at least 4 subdivisions of receptor described. The 5-HT$_1$ receptor has been subdivided into types A, B,

C, and D. Ondansetron acts on the 5-HT$_3$ receptor. 5-HT effects on coronary vasculature depend on the concentration and type of receptor present.

Ref: British Journal of Anaesthesia 1994: 73; 395-407

ANSWER   89

A. TRUE   B. TRUE   C. FALSE   D. FALSE   E. TRUE

The seizures are usually focal, progressing to tonic/clonic convulsions. They have a high (30%) mortality. Hypokalaemia is common.

ANSWER   90

A. TRUE   B. FALSE   C. TRUE   D. TRUE   E. FALSE

The hepatic clearance of a drug is controlled by two independent variables:

1 Hepatic Blood Flow (Qh)

2 The intrinsic ability of the liver to metabolize the drug (Cl int)

For many drugs eg thiopentone and diazepam Cl int << Qh; therefore hepatic clearance = Cl int.

Drugs such as these have a low extraction ratio and hepatic clearance is largely independent of hepatic blood flow. In fact, an increase in hepatic blood flow leads to a decrease in the extraction ratio. Their clearance may be increased by enzyme induction.Drugs with a high intrinsic clearance eg lignocaine, opioids, etomidate, and propofol have a hepatic clearance dependent on hepatic blood flow. They are unaffected by enzyme induction because of the already high extraction ratio. If the drug is given orally it is subject to a high first-pass metabolism in the liver.

Ref: Nimmo, Rowbotham, Smith. Anaesthesia, Blackwell, chapter 15

Exam 3

QUESTION 1

The following statements are true about digoxin

A. 75% of the oral dose is absorbed
B. 50% is bound to plasma proteins
C. Most is excreted unchanged in the urine
D. Hyperkalaemia may cause raised serum levels of digoxin
E. Toxicity may result in complete heart block

QUESTION 2

Restrictive lung disease is characterized by

A. A fall in FEV_1
B. A fall in arterial PO_2
C. A fall in FEV_1/FVC ratio
D. Carbon dioxide retention
E. A fall in vital capacity

QUESTION 3

The following serum concentrations are normal

A. A phosphate of 3.2 mmol/l
B. A magnesium of 2.25 mmol/l
C. A bilirubin of 12 mmol/l
D. A fasting glucose of 10 mmol/l
E. An albumin of 40 g/dl

QUESTION 4

Concerning drug dose and response

A. A plot of % response against drug concentration gives a sigmoid shape
B. Antagonists must have a higher receptor affinity than agonists
C. Intrinsic activity determines maximal response
D. Maximal response occurs only when all receptor sites are occupied
E. Partial agonism implies low receptor affinity

QUESTION 5

The following may lead to an increased anion gap

A. 0.9% Saline
B. Aspirin
C. Blood transfusion
D. Sodium nitroprusside
E. Methanol

QUESTION 6

Peripheral nerve

A. A-alpha fibres have a conduction velocity of 70-120 m/s
B. B fibres are unmyelinated
C. A-beta fibres convey afferent touch stimuli
D. Unmyelinated fibres can transmit at only 20 m/s
E. Conduction velocity is dependent upon nerve fibre diameter

QUESTION 7

The following are early signs of inadvertent oesophageal intubation

A. ST depression on electrocardiogram (ECG)
B. Bradycardia
C. Absence of waveform on capnograph
D. Absence of breath sounds on auscultation of lung apices
E. Oxyhaemoglobin desaturation detected on pulse oximetry

QUESTION 8

Student's t-test

A. Is so named because it is suitable for use by undergraduates
B. Can only be used for normally-distributed data
C. Can be used to compare one group before and after treatment as well as to compare two groups
D. Creates a value for t which indicates significance
E. Might be used to compare groups of data measuring blood pressure

QUESTION 9

During the explosive phase of a cough

A. Intra-pleural pressure of 90 mmHg may be produced
B. Cerebral perfusion pressure is reduced
C. There is a reduction in venous return
D. The airways narrow
E. The diaphragm contracts

QUESTION 10

In chronic anaemia

A. The O_2 dissociation curve is shifted to the left
B. Cyanosis is relatively easy to detect
C. Chemoreceptor stimulation is increased
D. Oxygen tension of arterial blood is unchanged
E. Blood volume is maintained by haemodilution

QUESTION 11

Isoprenaline

A. Is cardioselective
B. Decreases peripheral vascular resistance
C. Is equipotent with adrenaline
D. May decrease mean arterial pressure
E. Has a significant effect on alpha receptors

QUESTION 12

Diathermy safety

A. Ohm's law states that voltage = current x resistance
B. Diathermy works because there is a high current density at the active electrode
C. The heat energy produced by cautery is proportional to the current at the tip of the active electrode
D. Bipolar diathermy requires a passive electrode ('diathermy plate')
E. Poor contact of the passive electrode ('diathermy plate') may lead to inadvertent patient burns

QUESTION 13

The following drugs have a pKa greater than physiological pH

A. Salicylic acid
B. Diazepam
C. Lignocaine
D. Bupivacaine
E. Thiopentone

QUESTION 14

The following may lead to delivery of an inaccurately high concentration of anaesthetic agent

A. Pumping effect
B. Fall in the temperature of the anaesthetic agent
C. Low flows (500 ml/min)
D. Use of isoflurane in a halothane vaporiser
E. Turning a Tec 4 vaporiser upside down before use

QUESTION 15

The following are examples of physiological antagonism

A. Morphine and naloxone
B. Fentanyl and doxapram
C. Morphine and pentazocine
D. Ritodrine and syntocinon
E. Frusemide and amiloride

QUESTION 16

The rate of diffusion of a drug across a membrane is dependent upon

A. The drug concentration gradient across the membrane
B. Fick's Law
C. Dalton's Law
D. The surface area of the membrane
E. The degree of ionization of the drug

QUESTION 17

Insulin

A. Is synthesized in the endoplasmic reticulum of the beta cells
B. Has a half life of approximately two hours
C. Receptors are decreased in number with uraemia
D. Receptor affinity is decreased with acidosis
E. Decreases lipogenesis and glycogenesis in the liver

QUESTION 18

Halothane hepatitis

A. Occurs more commonly in males
B. Has a mortality of about 30%
C. Occurs with a maximum susceptibility when there has been about one month between exposures
D. Occurs following about 1 in 10000 cases of multiple administration of halothane
E. Has an onset most commonly beginning about 2 weeks after exposure

QUESTION 19

Ketorolac

A. Is an acetic acid
B. Has an analgesic potency similar to that of indomethacin
C. Following intramuscular injection has an analgesic effect lasting approximately 12 hours
D. Has no significant anti-pyretic action
E. Is approved for oral, intramuscular and intravenous administration

QUESTION 20

Nitrous oxide

A. Was discovered by Humphry Davy in 1772
B. Has been available in metal cylinders since the 1860's
C. Supports combustion
D. Is manufactured by heating ammonium nitrate to 350°C
E. Has a solubility in blood similar to that of desflurane

QUESTION 21

Dopexamine hydrochloride

A. Is a dobutamine analogue
B. Has significant alpha-adrenoceptor activity at higher doses
C. Acts mainly at beta-1 receptors to produce rises in cardiac output
D. Has been shown in many trials to reduce the incidence of acute renal failure in high risk surgical patients
E. Is thought to improve splanchnic blood flow

QUESTION 22

Concerning chronic pain

A. Allodynia is increased pain from a normally painful stimulus
B. Hyperalgesia is pain from a stimulus that is not normally painful
C. Hyperaesthesia includes allodynia and hyperalgesia
D. Dysaesthesia includes allodynia and hyperalgesia
E. Allodynia and hyperalgesia mean the same

QUESTION 23

The action of pancuronium is potentiated by

A. Renal failure
B. Hyperkalaemia
C. Hypomagnesaemia
D. Erythromicin
E. Isoflurane

QUESTION 24

In the eye

A. Contraction of the ciliary muscle flattens the lens
B. IgA is secreted in tears
C. Normal intraocular pressure is about 10mmHg
D. An axial length of 27mm is suggestive of myopia
E. Production of aqueous humor is dependent on carbonic anhydrase

QUESTION 25

In the management of ventricular fibrillation (VF)

A. The first task is to intubate to secure the airway
B. In the adult a DC shock of 360 Joules should be used first
C. The first dose of adrenaline should be given after 6 DC shocks
D. This is a common form of cardiac arrest in children
E. Bicarbonate 100 ml 8.4% should be given after one unsuccessful attempt at cardioversion

QUESTION 26

Response to acute haemorrhage includes

A. Increased plasma protein synthesis
B. Increased ADH secretion
C. Increased interstitial fluid formation
D. Reduced cortisol secretion
E. Decreased pulse pressure

QUESTION 27

Secretion of gastric acid is

A. Reduced by proton-pump inhibitors
B. Increased by histamine
C. Increased by duodenal acidification
D. Increased by cholecystokinin
E. Reduced by somatostatin

QUESTION 28

Desmopressin (DDAVP)

A. Is a synthetic analogue of vasopressin with similar pharmacological effects
B. Increases levels of von Willebrand's factor
C. Shortens the bleeding time in uraemic patients
D. Given repeatedly will demonstrate tachyphylaxis
E. Is associated with hypertension secondary to vasoconstriction

QUESTION 29

The following statements about selective phosphodiesterase (PDE) inhibitors are true

A. Inhibition of isoenzyme family No. I effects a positive inotropic action
B. Inhibition of isoenzyme family No. III results in clinically important bronchodilatation
C. They improve cardiac performance but cause significant increases in myocardial oxygen consumption
D. Bradycardia is a common occurrence
E. There is a risk of systemic hypotension associated with their use as inotropic agents

QUESTION 30

Aprotinin

- **A.** Is a polypeptide
- **B.** Inhibits plasmin and kallikrein
- **C.** Is derived from bovine lung
- **D.** Is metabolised and eliminated by the kidney
- **E.** Can be used to decrease blood loss during cardiac surgery

QUESTION 31

Measuring cardiac output by thermodilution

- **A.** Is accurate and easily repeatable
- **B.** Involves measuring the integral of the temperature change over time
- **C.** The latent heat of vaporisation of the injectate is used in the calculations
- **D.** Is also known as the Fick technique
- **E.** Measurement may be inaccurate due to respiratory changes in pulmonary artery temperature

QUESTION 32

Hemisection of the spinal cord causes

- **A.** Contralateral paralysis
- **B.** Ipsilateral loss of proprioception
- **C.** Ipsilateral loss of pain sensation
- **D.** Contralateral loss of vibration sense
- **E** Contralateral loss of temperature sensation

QUESTION 33

Rocuronium

- **A.** Has a structure which differs from vecuronium at two positions
- **B.** Is 5 to 10 times less potent than vecuronium
- **C.** Produces adequate intubating conditions as rapidly as suxamethonium
- **D.** Should be avoided in liver disease
- **E.** Undergoes hepatobiliary elimination

QUESTION 34

Ketamine

- **A.** Is a derivative of phencyclidine
- **B.** Is a bronchodilator
- **C** Maintains blood pressure following induction due to a direct stimulant effect on the heart
- **D.** Causes a rise in the cerebral oxygen consumption
- **E.** Is an agonist at the NMDA receptor

QUESTION 35

Calcitonin

A. Is produced by the parafollicular cells of the thyroid gland

B. Is a peptide hormone

C. Is not detectable in the serum if calcium levels are below 2 mmol/l

D. Stimulates osteoclast activity

E. Causes an increase in smooth muscle tone

QUESTION 36

Naloxone

A. Is a respiratory stimulant

B. Is a selective mu-1 antagonist

C. Reverses opioid induced vomiting

D. Has the same duration of action as morphine

E. May precipitate acute opioid withdrawal in susceptible patients

QUESTION 37

The peak flowmeter

A. Needs to be able to measure up to about 100 l/min flow

B. Is a variable orifice meter

C. Consists of a piston or vane that is moved against the resistance of a spring

D. Is designed to measure flow on a breath-by-breath basis

E. Tends to over-read compared with a pneumotachograph

QUESTION 38

Bilirubin

A. Is produced in the liver as a by-product of haemoglobin breakdown

B. Is conjugated by glucuronyl transferase to a more lipid soluble form

C. Is converted to urobilinogen within the jejunum

D. Is re-absorbed enterohepatically only in its conjugated form

E. Binds poorly to albumin

QUESTION 39

The a-wave in the jugular venous pulse

A. Is caused by atrial filling during ventricular systole

B. Is elevated in atrial fibrillation

C. Is reduced in tricuspid stenosis

D. Is elevated in pulmonary hypertension

E. Occurs immediately after ventricular systole

QUESTION 40

Protamine

- A. Is a strongly basic protein
- B. Is given in a dose of approximately 1 mg for every 1000 units of heparin
- C. Is isolated from bovine lung
- D. Combines with antithrombin III to displace heparin and thereby reverse anticoagulation
- E. Can result in flushing, hypotension and bronchoconstriction after intravenous administration

QUESTION 41

Saliva

- A. Its ionic composition depends on its flow rate
- B. Is hypertonic
- C. Its ionic composition depends on aldosterone
- D. Its secretion is easily conditioned
- E. About 1500 ml are secreted per day in a healthy adult

QUESTION 42

Ketone body formation

- A. Is increasd by a relative deficiency of oxaloacetic acid in the citric acid cycle
- B. Is increased by a high-fat, low-carbohydrate diet
- C. Leads to the presence of acetone in urine and expired air
- D. Is accompanied by condensation of acetyl-CoA units to form acetoacetyl-CoA
- E. Is increased by glucagon

QUESTION 43

2,3-Diphosphoglycerate concentration in red blood cells

- A. Rises acutely following exercise
- B. Is increased by growth hormone and thyroid hormones
- C. Does not affect the P_{50} of adult haemoglobin
- D. Is increased by a rise in blood pH
- E. Is reduced in the presence of decreased red cell glycolysis

QUESTION 44

A disposable endotracheal tube

- A. Is described by its external diameter
- B. Is marked with a code showing the place and date of manufacture
- C. Is visible on a radiograph
- D. Has a 15 mm connector for attachment to the anaesthetic circuit
- E. Has a cuff that is impervious to gases

QUESTION 45

The Fleisch Pneumotachograph

A. Is constant pressure flowmeter
B. Is not useful for breath-to-breath measurements
C. Is designed to measure laminar flow
D. Uses a pressure transducer to measure flow
E. Becomes inaccurate because condensation is common

QUESTION 46

Insulin

A. Is composed of two chains, alpha and beta
B. Is produced from a single chain precursor
C. Has an elimination half-life after intravenous injection of about an hour
D. Mostly circulates as free hormone
E. Is metabolised in the kidneys and liver by a proteolytic enzyme

QUESTION 47

Clonidine

A. Is a selective partial agonist for the alpha-2- adrenoceptor with a ratio of approximately 20:1 (alpha-2:alpha-1)
B. Is rapidly absorbed when given orally
C. When given as premedication, it reduces the MAC by up to 90%
D. Following discontinuation after prolonged use as an antihypertensive, there may be rebound hypertension
E. Has an antidiuretic effect in humans

QUESTION 48

Acetylcholine

A. Is the neurotransmitter at all autonomic preganglionic nerve endings
B. Is the neurotransmitter at all parasympathetic postganglionic nerve endings
C. Is generated from choline synthesized within the axoplasm
D. Raises the membrane permeability to sodium and calcium in the heart
E. Is released in quanta of approximately 4000 molecules per vesicle

QUESTION 49

Total lung compliance

A. Is slightly greater when measured during deflation rather than inflation
B. Is the pressure difference required to achieve a unit of air flow
C. Is decreased in the presence of interstitial pulmonary fibrosis
D. Is increased in the presence of emphysema
E. Will be approximately halved following endobronchial intubation

QUESTION 50

The Chi squared test

A. Is the sum of: (observed – expected) squared, divided by the expected frequencies
B. Is used for analysing derived statistics
C. Is suitable for data of a small sample size
D. Requires a correction for the number of degrees of freedom
E. Will have four degrees of freedom for a two by two table.

QUESTION 51

Concerning fetal haemoglobin

A. The molecule comprises two alpha chains and two delta chains
B. It is normally 80% replaced by HbA_2 at three months of age
C. It can persist through life
D. It contains more amino acids than adult haemoglobin
E. It strongly binds 2,3DPG

QUESTION 52

Concerning the metabolism of lignocaine

A. It is extensively metabolised by the liver
B. It undergoes oxidation followed by hydrolysis
C. Metabolism is decreased in cardiac failure
D. Metabolites accumulate in the presence of renal failure
E. It is metabolised more rapidly than prilocaine

QUESTION 53

In the management of an acute head injury

A. Steroids are useful in reducing cerebral oedema
B. Lumbar puncture should be used for determination of intracranial pressure (ICP)
C. Amnesia is an indication for computerised axial tomography of the brain (CT)
D. Where skull fracture and lowered level of consciousness are both present, the risk of intracranial haematoma is 1:4
E. Hartmann's solution should be avoided

QUESTION 54

Normal arterial pH is

A. Associated with an hydrogen ion concentration of 40 mmol/l
B. Maintained by excreting approximately 60 mmol hydrogen ions per day
C. Maintained principally by intracellular buffering systems
D. Calculated from measured PCO2 and bicarbonate in blood gas analysers ·
E. Is slightly higher in the neonate than in the adult

QUESTION 55

The following cause a rise in the end-tidal carbon dioxide level (assuming constant ventilation)

A. Hypothermia
B. Malignant hyperpyrexia
C. Pulmonary embolus
D. Disconnection of the inner tube of a Bain circuit
E. Failure of the endotracheal tube cuff

QUESTION 56

Labetolol

A. Acts on alpha and beta receptors with equal affinity
B. May cause retrograde ejaculation by its alpha blocking action
C. Has no intrinsic sympathomimetic activity (ISA)
D. Causes significant postural hypotension
E. Is contraindicated in pregnancy because it causes fetal bradycardia

QUESTION 57

For anti-inflammatory (glucocorticoid) activity prednisolone 5 mg is equivalent to

A. Hydrocortisone 100 mg
B. Methylprednisolone 4 mg
C. Dexamethasone 7.5 mg
D. Fludrocortisone 100 mg
E. Triamcinolone 4 mg

QUESTION 58

Concerning muscular diseases

A. The Guillain-Barre syndrome is an acute post-infective polyneuropathy
B. Muscular dystrophy spares cardiac muscle
C. Myasthenia gravis is associated with pulmonary malignancy
D. Neuromuscular blockade is hazardous
E. Edrophonium can relieve myasthenia gravis

QUESTION 59

Cylinders

A. Of nitrous oxide are marked with a tare weight
B. Of Entonox are filled to 93 bar (approx, at room temperature)
C. Of carbon dioxide are normally size F in anaesthetic use
D. Of size E may contain 680 litres of oxygen
E. Of Entonox should be stored vertically

QUESTION 60

When using clinical measuring devices

A. Ideally they should be critically damped
B. Oscilloscopic monitors exhibit arc distortion
C. Tangent error is a type of non-linearity
D. The resonant frequency should be low
E. A pen recorder will tend to show hysteresis error

QUESTION 61

The following hormones are peptides

A. Calcitonin
B. Oxytocin
C. ACTH
D. TSH
E. Erythropoietin

QUESTION 62

Vancomycin

A. Is effective against Gram negative aerobic organisms
B. Penetrates the CSF poorly
C. Is well absorbed orally
D. Can be associated with profound hypotension during intravenous administration
E. Inhibits bacterial cell wall synthesis

QUESTION 63

The following receive only sympathetic innervation

A. Lacrimal glands
B. Piloerector muscles
C. Adipose tissue
D. Juxtaglomerular apparatus
E. Pupils

QUESTION 64

The following cause vasodilatation of skeletal muscle blood vessels

A. Hydrogen ions
B. Potassium ions
C. Adenosine
D. Hyperthermia
E. Stimulation of sympathetic cholinergic fibres

QUESTION 65

In ketoacidotic diabetic coma

A. Large volume administration of dextrose-containing solutions are required in resuscitation
B. Potassium supplementation will be required
C. The hourly insulin requirement can be calculated by dividing the daily requirement by 24
D. Bicarbonate therapy is needed with an arterial pH above 7.0
E. Artificial ventilation may be required

QUESTION 66

The following hormones are secreted by the placenta

A. Renin
B. Prolactin
C. Cortisol
D. Progesterone
E. Vasopressin

QUESTION 67

Intravenous regional anaesthesia (Bier's block)

A. Can safely be performed using 0.25% bupivacaine without adrenaline
B. Provides good quality postoperative analgesia
C. Depends on the use of a double-cuff tourniquet inflated to 50 mmHg above systolic pressure
D. The tourniquet can safely be deflated 20 minutes after injection
E. An advantage of the technique is that it can be employed by unsupervised casualty officers

QUESTION 68

Humidity

A. Absolute humidity = volume of water vapour in unit volume of air at specified pressure & temperature
B. Relative humidity = partial pressure of water vapour divided by the SVP of water at specified temperature
C. Absolute humidity can be measured by a Regnault's hygrometer
D. The Regnault's hygrometer relies on evaporation
E. The Regnault's hygrometer relies on condensation

QUESTION 69

Trimetaphan

A. Blocks parasympathetic ganglia to produce hypotension
B. Relaxes both resistance and capacitance vessels
C. Is inactivated by plasma cholinesterase
D. Has a half-life of about 30 minutes
E. May cause histamine release

QUESTION 70

Medical lasers

A. Laser is an acronym for Light Amplification by Stimulated Emission of Radiation
B. Retinal surgery may be performed by using carbon dioxide lasers
C. Matt-surfaced instruments should be used
D. The light produced is parallel, multi-phasic and of specific wavelength
E. The light is normally focused at about 25-50mm from the tip of the probe

QUESTION 71

Electrical equipment

A. The risk of ventricular fibrillation is greatest if the AC current has a frequency of about 50 Hz
B. Should conform to BS5724 for use in theatre
C. If used with intra-cardiac leads may lead to ventricular fibrillation at currents of 10 μA
D. If battery-operated will not cause microshock
E. If used in theatre the circuit in contact with the patient must be earthed

QUESTION 72

Oxytocin

A. Stimulates production of milk
B. Stimulates milk ejection
C. Release is stimulated by dilatation of the cervix
D. Is synthesized in the anterior pituitary
E. Produces more powerful uterine contraction in the presence of progesterone

QUESTION 73

Concerning the cardiac cycle

A. The aortic valve opens at the start of ventricular systole
B. The aortic valve closes at the end of ventricular systole
C. The mitral valve closes at the start of ventricular systole
D. Carotid pressure is highest at the start of ventricular systole
E. Left ventricular volume is lowest when the mitral valve opens

QUESTION 74

The following are true concerning standard (unfractionated) heparin

A. Hypersensitivity reactions are common
B. The best monitor of full anticoagulation is the activated partial thromboplastin time
C. Thrombocytopenia is a recognised complication
D. Long term use carries a risk of alopecia
E. It is inactivated by desulphation in the reticuloendothelial system

QUESTION 75

Considering postoperative complications

A. Deep vein thrombosis (DVT) is common after lower limb surgery
B. The commonest cause of chest pain on the third postoperative day is a pulmonary embolism
C. Wound abscess formation is suggested by fever and an elevated white cell count on the sixth postoperative day
D. Postoperative myocardial infarction (MI) occurs in at least 5% of patients who have had an MI in the previous three months
E. Postoperative myocardial infarction carries a 25% mortality

QUESTION 76

Plasma cholinesterase

A. Acquired deficiencies of the enzyme in genotypically normal patients prolongs suxamethonium activity for several hours
B. The commonest genotype for cholinesterase activity is E1u E1u
C. Deficiency occurs in pregnancy
D. Homozygotes always experience a prolonged suxamethonium block
E. Patients who are homozygotes for the fluoride resistant gene have a near normal dibucaine number

QUESTION 77

Trials and research

A. Ethical committee approval is invariably required for audit projects
B. The Declaration of Helsinki deals with the safeguarding of patients undergoing clinical trials
C. Consent of patients is not needed if a clear benefit from the control treatment is known
D. Randomisation of subjects is desirable
E. Double blinding means neither the doctor nor the statistician are aware of treatment groups

QUESTION 78

If the haematocrit is 40% and plasma volume is 3 litres

A. Total blood volume = 4000 ml
B. The patient's body weight should be approximately 60 kg
C. The patient is probably female
D. Plasma viscosity will be significantly elevated
E. A total blood volume of 85 ml/kg is a reasonable estimate

QUESTION 79

The following statements are true

A. Correlation indicates causation
B. The power of a study is 1 minus the alpha error
C. The standard error of the mean is the standard deviation divided by the number in the sample
D. A sample that is not normally distributed may be transformed into a Gaussian distribution
E. Ordinal data may be described statistically by the use of median and percentiles

QUESTION 80

Concerning the ECG

A. The P-R interval represents the total time taken for atrial depolarisation
B. The Q-T interval is normally less than or equal to 0.49 s
C. The formula for corrected Q-T in tachycardia is Q-T divided by the R-R interval squared
D. The normal range for the P-R interval is 0.06 to 0.10 s
E. QRS greater than 0.10 s represents conduction delay

QUESTION 81

Epiglottitis

A. Is commonest in children between six months and three years
B. There may be no systemic upset in the child
C. Cannulation is mandatory before attempting to control the airway
D. Staphylococcus is the usual causative organism
E. Intubation for 24 hours is usual

QUESTION 82

Blood-gas analysis

A. The base excess is the amount of strong acid required to return the pH of 1 litre of blood to 7.40 at a PCO_2 of 5.3 kPa and 37°C

B. Too much heparinised saline tends to cause a falsely low reading of the $PaCO_2$

C. Too much heparin tends to cause a falsely low reading of potassium concentration

D. Measurement of oxygen content is provided by routine blood gas analysis

E. Prolonged storage at 4°C may lead to a falsely low value for PaO_2

QUESTION 83

The following are true

A. An ECG can be broken down into a set of sine waves

B. Two sine waves 180° out of phase will cancel each other out

C. X-rays travel slower than light

D. In the EEG beta waves have a higher frequency than alpha waves

E. In the EEG delta waves have a higher frequency than alpha waves

QUESTION 84

Recognised methods of measuring anaesthetic vapour concentration include

A. Mass spectrometry

B. Ultraviolet light absorption

C. Thermal conductivity

D. Paramagnetism

E. Raman scattering

QUESTION 85

Myocardial infarction is associated with

A. Guillain-Barre syndrome

B. Uncontrolled hypertension

C. Anaesthesia within one year of previous infarction

D. Isoflurane anaesthesia and the coronary steal syndrome

E. Sepsis

QUESTION 86

Methohexitone

A. When made up as a 1% solution is only stable at room temperature for about 24 hours

B. Undergoes greater hepatic clearance than thiopentone

C. Is associated with involuntary movements following intravenous administration

D. Is more potent than thiopentone.

E. Decreases cerebral blood volume by causing cerebral vasoconstriction

QUESTION 87

Sevoflurane

A. Is a hexafluoroisopropyl fluoromethyl ether
B. Undergoes minimal biotransformation in the liver to produce inorganic fluoride ions
C. Releases carbon monoxide when in contact with soda lime
D. Has a lower SVP than isoflurane
E. Has a blood:gas partition coefficient approximately half that of isoflurane

QUESTION 88

Concerning cardiac pacemakers

A. Suxamethonium may cause pacemaker inhibition
B. Unipolar diathermy is safe in the presence of a pacemaker
C. Bipolar diathermy is safe in the presence of a pacemaker
D. A "V V I" pacemaker indicates that it is the ventricle which is being paced
E. Symptomatic first degree heart block is an indication for temporary pacing

QUESTION 89

Statistical definition

A. T represents the mean difference divided by the standard error
B. Variance is the sum of the differences divided by the degrees of freedom
C. Standard error of the mean is the square root of the variance
D. Standard deviation is the standard error of the mean divided by the square root of the number observed
E. A normal distribution is one where the mean, mode and median are the same

QUESTION 90

In calculating lung volumes

A. Anatomical dead space may be estimated using the Bohr equation
B. Vd/Vt is normally 0.3 at rest
C. Functional residual capacity cannot be measured directly
D. Changes in expired nitrogen concentration may be used to determine closing volume
E. Changes in expired nitrogen concentration may be used to determine residual volume

Exam 3: Answers

ANSWER 1

A. TRUE   B. FALSE   C.TRUE   D. FALSE   E. TRUE

There is insignificant binding to plasma proteins. Hypokalaemia may precipitate digitalis toxicity. All forms of heart block have been recorded in digitalis toxicity.

ANSWER 2

A. TRUE   B. TRUE   C. FALSE   D. FALSE   E. TRUE

Restrictive lung disease may be characterized by parenchymal or chest wall changes. Lung diseases include sarcoidosis and fibrosing alveolitis, while lesions of the chest wall include kyphoscoliosis and ankylosing spondylitis. Pulmonary function tests generally reveal a decrease in both FEV_1 and FVC with a normal FEV_1/FVC ratio. TLC and FRC will be reduced as will compliance. Small airway closure occurs during tidal ventilation causing shunting and hypoxaemia, but $PaCO_2$ is likely to be unaffected. The work of breathing is increased and ability to cough is impaired.

Ref: Aitkenhead, Smith. Textbook of Anaesthesia. Churchill Livingstone, Ch41

ANSWER 3

A. FALSE   B. FALSE   C. FALSE   D. FALSE   E. FALSE

Typical normal ranges are: Phosphate 0.8-1.4 mmol/l (elevated in renal failure); Magnesium 0.7-1.0 mmol/l (Calcium is 2.1-2.6 mmol/l); Bilirubin 5-17 mcmol/l; Glucose 3.3-6.7 mmol/l; Albumin 35-50 g/l.

ANSWER 4

A. FALSE   B. FALSE   C. TRUE   D. FALSE   E. FALSE

Dose response curves are normally plotted as % response against LOG drug concentration. The resultant graph is sigmoid shaped. A drug with high affinity and high intrinsic activity is an agonist. A drug with high affinity but no intrinsic activity will act as an antagonist, however displacement of an agonist also depends on the relative concentrations of the two drugs at the receptor sites. Partial agonism may be displayed by a drug with low intrinsic activity, but it may well have high receptor affinity making it difficult to antagonize. A maximal response may be achieved by activation of a small proportion of receptor sites (eg the NMJ)

Ref: Aitkenhead & Smith. Textbook of Anaesthesia.

ANSWER 5

A. FALSE   B. TRUE   C. TRUE   D. TRUE   E. TRUE

The anion gap = $(Na + K)-(Cl+ HCO_3)$
Normal range = 12 +/- 2 mEq/l

It reflects the presence of anions other than chloride and bicarbonate that counterbalance the cationic charge of sodium. An increase is seen when $HCO3$ is replaced by organic (lactate, keto acids) or inorganic (sulphate, phosphate) acids, or by the presence of toxins (salicylate, glycolate, formate). When it exceeds 30 mEq/l it is almost always indicative of organic acid acidosis.

INCREASED ANION GAP

Lactic acidosis
Renal failure
Ketoacidosis (DM, starvation)
Toxins (ethylene glycol, methanol, salicylates)
Sodium nitroprussideAcid infusion (ACD blood, fructose)

Ref: Nunn, Utting, Brown. General Anaesthesia. Butterworths.

ANSWER 6

A. TRUE   B. FALSE   C. TRUE   D. FALSE   E. TRUE

Nerve fibre diameter determines cross-sectional area which is inversely related to longitudinal resistance of the axon. C fibres are unmyelinated.
A-alpha = muscle afferents & efferents = 70-120 m/s.
A-beta = touch afferents = 30-70 m/s.
A-gamma = muscle spindle efferents = 15-30 m/s.
A-delta = temp & fast pain = 12-30 m/s.
B = sympathetic preganglionic = 3-15 m/s.
C = sympathetic postganglionic & slow pain = 0.5-2 m/s.
Diameters decrease through the group.

Ref: Despopoulos A, Silbernagl S. Color Atlas of Physiology, 22-49

ANSWER 7

A. FALSE   B. FALSE   C. TRUE   D. FALSE   E. FALSE

Especially if preceded by preoxygenation, signs of hypoxia such as desaturation, bradycardia and ECG changes are late warnings. Capnography is the gold standard but careful auscultation is also helpful in confirming correct placement, although it cannot reliably detect oesophageal placement.

ANSWER 8

A. FALSE   B. TRUE   C. TRUE   D. FALSE   E. TRUE

Student was the pseudonym for one William Gosset who was a chemist. The test is used for interval scale, normally distributed data such as blood pressure; the t value obtained does not itself indicate significance, but has to be read in a table next to the degrees of freedom and a p value obtained for this to be the case. The paired t-test is used to compare one group before and after treatment; the unpaired test is used to compare two groups.

ANSWER 9

A. TRUE   **B. TRUE**   **C. TRUE**   **D. TRUE**   **E. FALSE**

A deep inspiration is followed by forceful expiration against a closed glottis which increases intra-thoracic pressure along with central venous pressure. The glottis opens suddenly allowing forceful expiration through narrowed airways thus expelling debris. The diaphragm relaxes.

Ref: Nunn JF. Applied Respiratory Physiology. Butterworth-Heinemann

ANSWER 10

A. FALSE   **B. FALSE**   **C. FALSE**   **D. TRUE**   **E. TRUE**

In chronic anaemia there is increased 2,3DPG, therefore the O_2 dissociation curve is shifted to the right. Cyanosis is difficult to detect as there is less total deoxygenated haemoglobin to produce discolouration for any level of desaturation. Chemoreceptors respond to oxygen tension not content.

Ref: Yentis, Hirsch, Smith. Anaesthesia A to Z. Butterworth-Heinemann

ANSWER 11

A. FALSE   **B. TRUE**   **C. FALSE**   **D. TRUE**   **E. FALSE**

Isoprenaline is a synthetic catecholamine which is more potent than adrenaline. It acts on beta-1 and beta-2 receptors to produce an increase in cardiac output, tachycardia, and a fall in peripheral resistance which may cause a fall in mean arterial blood pressure. It is a powerful positive inotrope and chronotrope whose actions are mediated by membrane bound adenlyate cyclase. It has not activity at alpha receptors.

ANSWER 12

A. TRUE   **B. TRUE**   **C. FALSE**   **D. FALSE**   **E. TRUE**

Diathermy relies on generation of heat energy from electrical energy. Ohm's law states that voltage = current x resistance (V=IR). The heat energy produced = $(current)^2$ x resistance ($E=I^2R$). At the active electrode there is a high current density due to the small area of the electrode. This leads to the heat energy and cautery. The passive electrode ('diathermy plate') used with unipolar diathermy has a large area and so the current density (and hence the heat produced) is small. However if the contact is poor then either there is a reduced area of contact (with a higher current density) or increased resistance. As $E=I^2R$ both these faults lead to an increased risk of burning. Bipolar diathermy does not have a passive electrode, and the current passes from an active electrode to a return electrode; these are the two blades of the diathermy forceps

Ref: Faust RJ (ed). Anesthesiology Review, 2nd edn. Churchill Livingstone, 1994

ANSWER 13

A. FALSE   **B. FALSE**   **C. TRUE**   **D. TRUE**   **E. TRUE**

The pKa is the negative logarithm of the dissociation constant of an acid or the conjugate acid of a base, such that:

For an acid:- pH = pKa + log (ionized / unionized)

For a base:- pH = pKa + log (unionized / ionized)

In practice it is the pH at which 50% ionization occurs. If the pH is lower than the pKa, weak bases will tend to dissociate more, and weak acids will tend to become less ionized (vice versa at higher pH).

Salicylic acid pKa = 3 (therefore 9% ionized at pH=2, and 99.99% ionized at pH=7.4) hence alkalinization of urine promotes excretion by preventing tubular reabsorption of the ionized form in the nephron.

Diazepam pKa = 3.5 (basic drug)

Lignocaine pKa = 7.9

Bupivacaine pKa = 8.1 (all the commonly used local agents are basic drugs with pKa>7.4)

Thiopentone pKa = 7.6 (61% unionized at pH 7.4)

Methohexitone pKa = 7.9 (75% unionized at pH 7.4) All the barbiturates are weak acids

Ref: Nunn, Utting, Brown. General Anaesthesia. Butterworths.

ANSWER 14

A. TRUE   B. FALSE   C. TRUE   D. FALSE   E. FALSE

Vaporisers may become inaccurate if there is a change in the temperature of the agent (delivering a lower concentration), or at low flows (higher concentration). Pumping effect increases vaporisation due to the back-and-forth movement of the gas during the action of ventilators such as the Manley. Halothane and isoflurane have the same boiling point, so they could be used interchangeably (though this is not recommended). The Tec 4 vaporisers are able to withstand tilt up to 180° with no ill effects.

Ref: Davey A, Moyle JTB, Ward CS. Ward's Anaesthetic Equipment, 3rd edn. W.B. Saunders, 1992

ANSWER 15

A. FALSE   B. TRUE   C. FALSE   D. TRUE   E. TRUE

Morphine and naloxone are acting at the same receptor, thus this is a pharmacological antagonism. Morphine and pentazocine are not acting on opposing physiological mechanisms.

ANSWER 16

A. TRUE   B. TRUE   C. FALSE   D. TRUE   E. TRUE

Membranes tend to separate aqueous phases. Drug diffusion only occurs if a concentration gradient exists. It proceeds until the concentrations are equal. Rate of transfer obeys Fick's Law of diffusion:

$X/T = K.A.(C_1-C_2)/D$

X/T = Mass of drug divided by time

K = Drug diffusion coefficient (Affected by partition coefficient, molecular weight, and drug pKa)

A   = Membrane surface area

D = Membrane thickness

C_1-C_2 = Concentration gradient

Dalton's Law of partial pressures states that the pressure exerted by a mixture of gases or vapours enclosed in a given space, is equal to the sum of the pressures which each gas would exert if it alone were present.

Ref: Nimmo, Rowbotham, Smith. Anaesthesia, Blackwell, chapter 15

ANSWER 17

A. TRUE   B. FALSE   C. TRUE   D. TRUE   E. FALSE

Insulin has a half life of 10-30 min. Lipogenesis is stimulated in liver and fat tissues. Glycogenesis is stimulated in liver and muscle.

Ref: Despopoulos A, Silbernagl S. Color Atlas of Physiology. 232-270.

ANSWER 18

A. FALSE   B. FALSE   C. TRUE   D. FALSE   E. FALSE

Halothane hepatitis occurs more commonly in females. It has a mortality of 50-80%. It occurs after 1 in 3500 multiple administrations, and the onset is usually about 5 days after exposure.

Ref: Hepatoxicity of volatile anaesthetics. British Journal of Anaesthesia 1993; 70: 339-348

ANSWER 19

A. TRUE   B. FALSE   C. FALSE   D. FALSE   E. TRUE

Ketorolac is an NSAID with an analgesic potency six times that of indomethacin and an antipyretic action twenty times that of aspirin. Its anti-inflammatory potency is between that of naproxen and indomethacin. After intramuscular injection, analgesia occurs within 30 minutes, with a peak at 1-2 hours, and a duration of approximately 6 hours.

ANSWER 20

A. FALSE   B. TRUE   C. TRUE   D. FALSE   E. TRUE

Nitrous oxide was discovered by Priestley in 1772. It was available as a compressed gas in metal cylinders in London from 1868. Ammonium nitrate is heated to 270°C. Above 290°C the reaction is explosive. Its blood:gas partition coefficient (0.47) is similar to that of desflurane (0.42).

PHYSICAL:

  BP -88°C, CT 36.5°C, CP 71.7 atm, MAC 105, BG sol coeff 0.47, SG 1.53

ANSWER 21

A. FALSE   B. FALSE   C. FALSE   D. FALSE   E. TRUE

Dopexamine is an analogue of dopamine. It acts mainly at beta-2 and DA-1/DA-2 receptors. It has no alpha activity. It also inhibits uptake-1. Side effects include nausea, vomiting, hypokalaemia and hypoglycaemia. It is a weak positive inotrope but powerful splanchnic vasodilator reducing afterload. It has natiuretic and diuretic properties. There are no studies to support this.

Ref: Hinds, Watson. Intensive Care: A Concise Textbook. Saunders.

ANSWER 22

A. FALSE   B. FALSE   C. TRUE   D. TRUE   E. FALSE

Allodynia is pain from a stimulus that is not normally painful whereas hyperalgesia is increased pain from a normally painful stimulus, they are not the same. Hyperaesthesia is a broad term and means increased sensitivity to a sensory stimulus, whereas dysaesthesia is any abnormal unpleasant sensation, hence both of these include allodynia and hyperalgesia.

Ref: Yentis, Hirsch, Smith. Anaesthesia A to Z. Butterworth-Heinemann.

ANSWER 23

A. TRUE   B. FALSE   C. FALSE   D. FALSE   E. TRUE

The action of non depolarising muscle relaxants is potentiated by the following: Hypokalaemia, Hypermagnesaemia, Hypocalcaemia, Acidosis, Hypothermia, Volatile, and induction agents, Aminoglycoside antibiotics, Metronidazole.

Ref: Sasada, Smith. Drugs in Anaesthesia and Intensive Care

ANSWER 24

A. FALSE   B. TRUE   C. FALSE   D. TRUE   E. TRUE

The lens is supported by zonular fibres which apply tension that tends to flatten it, accommodating far vision at rest. Contraction of the ciliary muscle relaxes the tension of the zonular fibres allowing the lens to adopt a more spherical shape for near vision. Intraocular pressure is normally 15-22 mmHg. Axial length is increased with short-sightedness and a value >26mm would be compatible with myopia.

Ref: Despopoulos A, Silbernagl S. Color Atlas of Physiology. 300-315

ANSWER 25

A. FALSE   B. FALSE   C. FALSE   D. FALSE   E. FALSE

DC shock precedes intubation. The starting DC shock is 200 Joules in the adult. Adrenaline 1 mg is the first dose; 5 mg is given later. It is given after 3 shocks. VF is the commonest mode of arrest in the adult, children tend to bradyarrhythmias and asystole. Alkalising agents should not be used until three loops have been tried. You should ensure that you know all the protocols published by the ERC and that you are able to reproduce the algorithms.

Ref: European Resuscitation Council Guidelines

ANSWER 26

A. TRUE   B. TRUE   C. FALSE   D. FALSE   E. TRUE

Hydrostatic capillary pressure is reduced by a fall in systemic blood pressure and increased plasma protein synthesis increases colloid osmotic pressure; therefore fluid is encouraged to enter capillaries from the interstitium. Cortisol secretion is, as one would expect, increased.

Ref: Ganong WF. Review of Medical Physiology. Lange. Ch33.

ANSWER 27

A. TRUE   B. TRUE   C. FALSE   D. FALSE   E. TRUE

Duodenal acidification increases secretin secretion which reduces gastric acid secretion. Cholecystokinin reduces gastric acid secretion and reduces gastric emptying.

Ref: Ganong WF. Review of Medical Physiology. Lange.

ANSWER 28

A. FALSE   B. TRUE   C. TRUE   D. TRUE   E. FALSE

DDAVP has a longer lasting antidiuretic effect but lacks the vasoconstrictor effects of vasopressin. Its use is associated with hypotension, probably secondary to release of prostacyclin from endothelial cells. It may be given intranasally, orally or by injection. It may also be used to increase factor VIII and vWF in mild haemophilia and von Willibrand's disease.

Ref: Yentis, Hirsch, Smith. Anaesthesia A to Z. Butterworth-Heinemann

ANSWER 29

A. FALSE   B. FALSE   C. FALSE   D. FALSE   E. TRUE

Inhibition of isoenzyme family No. III results in positive inotropy. Bronchodilation does occur but not to a clinically significant degree. There is unchanged or even slightly reduced myocardial oxygen consumption as systemic vasodilation reduces left ventricular systolic wall tension. There is a reflex tachycardia. The hypotension seen is often very difficult to treat requiring volume loading and vasoconstrictor therapy.

Ref: British Journal of Anaesthesia 1992; 68: 293-302

ANSWER 30

A. TRUE   B. TRUE   C. TRUE   D. TRUE   E. TRUE

Aprotinin is a 58 amino acid polypeptide derived from bovine lung. In addition to inhibition of kallikrein and plasmin, aprotinin may decrease blood loss in cardiac surgery by helping to preserve platelet function. It has also been used in the management of pancreatitis and carcinoid syndrome.

ANSWER 31

A. TRUE   B. TRUE   C. FALSE   D. FALSE   E. TRUE

The thermodilution technique using a pulmonary artery catheter gives an accurate, easily repeatable measurement of cardiac output. The cardiac output is assessed by measuring the area under the curve of the temperature change recorded at the distal end of the catheter by a thermistor. this is the integral of the curve with respect to time. Calculation requires knowledge of the specific heat of the injectate and the blood (but not the latent heat of vaporisation). Errors may occur due to the pulmonary artery flow and temperature changes that occur with the respiratory cycle. The Fick technique measures cardiac output by measuring the arterio-venous difference of a specific gas (normally either oxygen or carbon dioxide) and its rate of uptake (or elimination) from the lungs.

Ref: Sykes MK, Vickers MD, Hull CJ. Principles of Measurement and Monitoring in Anaesthesia and Intensive Care, 3rd edn. Blackwell Scientific Publishers, 1991

ANSWER 32

A. FALSE   B. TRUE   C. FALSE   D. FALSE   E. TRUE

Brown-Sequard syndrome (hemisection of the spinal cord) causes ipsilateral paralysis and loss of proprioception, touch and vibration sensation, with contralateral loss of pain and temperature sensation.

Ref: Yentis, Hirsch, Smith. Anaesthesia A to Z. Butterworth-Heinemann.

ANSWER 33

A. FALSE **B. TRUE** **C. FALSE** **D. FALSE** **E. TRUE**

Rocuronium was developed from the vecuronium molecule and differs from it in four positions. It is 40-60 seconds slower than suxamethonium in producing intubating conditions. Although it is rapid in onset it has a duration of action similar to vecuronium. The lower potency of the drug appears to be related to its rapid onset of action, perhaps due to an increased concentration gradient created between plasma and NMJ. Like all the steroidal based neuromuscular blockers there is an element of hepatobilary excretion.

ANSWER 34

A. TRUE **B. TRUE** **C. FALSE** **D. TRUE** **E. FALSE**

The drug is a potent cardiovascular stimulant. This effect is mediated via a stimulation of the CNS with a resultant increase in sympathetic nervous system outflow rather than a direct myocardial effect. It should be used with caution in patients with ischaemic heart disease due to the increase in myocardial oxygen consumption.

ANSWER 35

A. TRUE **B. TRUE** **C. TRUE** **D. FALSE** **E. FALSE**

Calcitonin and PTH are both peptide hormones; 1,25-dihydroxycholecalciferol acts as a steroid hormone. Calcitonin is produced by the C cells or parafollicular cells within the thyroid gland. In hypercalcaemia the plasma concentration rises several fold. It lowers serum calcium by its action on bone, inhibiting the PTH mediated stimulation of osteoclasts and thereby increasing incorporation of calcium into bone matrix.

Ref: Despopoulos A, Silbernagl S. Color Atlas of Physiology, 232-271

ANSWER 36

A. FALSE **B. FALSE** **C. FALSE** **D. FALSE** **E. TRUE**

It reverses mu-receptor mediated respiratory depression. It acts preferentially at the mu receptor but also acts at the kappa and the delta receptors but not at the sigma receptor. The duration of action is shorter than that of morphine.

ANSWER 37

A. FALSE **B. TRUE** **C. TRUE** **D. FALSE** **E. FALSE**

Peak expiratory flow may be measured either with a Wright's respirometer or a piston device. Both are variable orifice devices that consist of a vane or piston that is moved by the incident air flow. This movement is resisted by a spring, and as the vane or piston moves it opens a channel in a progressive manner. The flowmeter should be able to measure up to about 1000 l/min peak flow. It is designed for single measurements, and because of the inertia of the spring tends to under-read when compared with the pneumotachograph.

Ref: Sykes MK, Vickers MD, Hull CJ. Principles of Measurement and Monitoring in Anaesthesia and Intensive Care, 3rd edn. Blackwell Scientific Publishers, 1991

ANSWER 38

A. FALSE   **B. FALSE**   **C. TRUE**   **D. FALSE**   **E. FALSE**

85% of bilirubin arises from the breakdown of RBCs. It is released by macrophages and is transported to the liver bound tightly to albumin. Free unconjugated bilirubin is poorly soluble in water but highly lipid soluble, rendering it centrally neurotoxic. Following hepatic uptake, it is conjugated to bilirubin glucuronide which is water-soluble, non-toxic, and actively secreted into bile canaliculi. 15% is reabsorbed enterohepatically, but only in the lipid-soluble unconjugated form. Urobilinogen (colourless) is formed both in the liver and the intestine. Further bacterial breakdown to stercobilinogen (colourless) is followed by partial oxidation to the pigmented urobilin or stercobilin found in the stools.

Ref: Despopoulos A, Silbernagl S. Color Atlas of Physiology, 216

ANSWER 39

A. FALSE   **B. FALSE**   **C. FALSE**   **D. TRUE**   **E. FALSE**

The a-wave is due to atrial contraction, and is therefore absent in AF. Large a-waves are seen in tricuspid stenosis and pulmonary hypertension.

Ref: Yentis, Hirsch, Smith. Anaesthesia A to Z. Butterworth-Heinemann

ANSWER 40

A. TRUE   **B. FALSE**   **C. FALSE**   **D. FALSE**   **E. TRUE**

Protamine is a mixture of cationic, basic low molecular weight proteins found in fish testes. It binds with acidic heparin to form a complex devoid of anticoagulant properties (a stable salt). 1 mg of protamine reverses the anticoagulant effect of 100 iu of heparin. Side effects include myocardial depression, bradycardia, pulmonary hypertension, histamine release, complement activation and anaphylactic reactions. These effects are more pronounced with rapid injection.

Ref: Yentis, Hirsch, Smith. Anaesthesia A to Z. Butterworth-Heinemann

ANSWER 41

A. TRUE   **B. FALSE**   **C. TRUE**   **D. TRUE**   **E. TRUE**

Saliva is hypotonic and its ionic composition depends on flow rate and aldosterone secretion. about 1500 ml per day are secreted by a healthy adult and its secretion is readily conditioned as proved in the famous experiments on dogs by Pavlov.

Ref: Ganong WF. Review of Medical Physiology, Lange

ANSWER 42

A. TRUE   **B. TRUE**   **C. TRUE**   **D. TRUE**   **E. TRUE**

Ketosis occurs in starvation, diabetes mellitus, and a high-fat & low-carbohydrate diet which all cause intracellular carbohydrate starvation. Insufficient oxaloacetic acid is formed to condense with acetyl-CoA (which builds up). Formation of acetoacetic acid leads to acetone and beta-hydroxybutyric acid formation.

Ref: Ganong WF. Review of Medical Physiology. Lange, Ch17

ANSWER 43

A. TRUE   B. TRUE   C. FALSE   D. TRUE   E. TRUE

2,3-DPG causes liberation of oxygen peripherally by binding to beta chains of the haemoglobin molecule. It is produced by glycolysis via the Embden-Meyerhof pathway.

Ref: Ganong WF. Review of Medical Physiology. Lange. Ch34.

ANSWER 44

A.FALSE   B. FALSE   C. TRUE   D. TRUE   E. FALSE

A standard disposable endotracheal tube is described by its internal diameter, and is marked with a code concerning implantation testing. The tube has a radio-opaque line and is fitted with an 'International 15' 15 mm connector. The cuff is not impervious to gases, so during prolonged anaesthesia there is a risk of increased cuff pressure due to absorption of nitrous oxide.

Ref: Davey A, Moyle JTB, Ward CS. Ward's Anaesthetic Equipment, 3rd edn. W.B. Saunders., 1992

ANSWER 45

A. FALSE   B. FALSE   C. TRUE   D. TRUE   E. FALSE

The Fleisch Pneumotachograph is a fast-responding constant orifice (variable pressure) transducer that relies on measuring the pressure difference across a fixed resistance. The resistance is provided by two corrugated strips of metal foil. The flow through the machine in its operating range is laminar. Condensation is prevented by a heating element that keeps the machine just above body temperature. Because of its fast response it is ideal for breath-to-breath measurements.

Ref: Wallis BA, Lunn JN. The measurement of gas flow and volume. In: Scurr C, Feldman S, Soni N (Eds) Scientific Foundations of Anaesthesia; The Basis of Intensive Care, 4th edn. Heinemann Medical Books, 1990, pp 104-114

ANSWER 46

A. FALSE   B. TRUE   C. FALSE   D. TRUE   E. TRUE

Insulin is produced from proinsulin, a polypeptide synthesised by the beta cells of the islets of Langerhans. It is composed of two chains, A and B, joined by three disulphide bonds. Its elimination half-life is about 10 minutes, but the pharmacological effect is more prolonged (30 to 60 minutes) due to binding to tissue receptors.

ANSWER 47

A. FALSE   B. TRUE   C. FALSE   D. TRUE   E. FALSE

The ratio is 200:1(the higher the affinity for the alpha-2 receptor the more efficacious the drug). Bioavailability is good. It does reduce MAC but only the highly selective drugs such as dexmemdetomidine have lowered anaesthetic requirements to this degree. It inhibits the release of ADH and causes an increase in the GFR.

Ref: Seminars in Anesthesia 1996; 15(1)

ANSWER 48

A. TRUE   B. TRUE   C. FALSE   D. FALSE   E. TRUE

An acetyl group from acetylcoenzyme A is transferred to choline in the presence of ChAT (choline acetyl transferase). However, choline cannot be synthesized within nerves and is accumulated from the ECF. 50% of the choline formed from ACh breakdown in the synaptic cleft is reabsorbed. ACh raises the membrane permeability to Na, K, and Ca in most tissues, but in the heart only K permeability is increased.

Ref: Despopoulos A, Silbernagl S. Color Atlas of Physiology. 50-59

ANSWER 49

A. TRUE   B. FALSE   C. TRUE   D. TRUE   E. TRUE

Resistance of the lung and chest is the pressure difference required to achieve a unit of air flow. Compliance is dependent on lung volume. A hysteresis compliance curve exists.

Ref: Ganong WF. Review of Medical Physiology. Lange. Ch34.

ANSWER 50

A. TRUE   B. FALSE   C. FALSE   D. TRUE   E. FALSE

The Chi squared test is used for the non-parametric analysis of nominal data comparing groups consisting of different subjects with different treatments. It is used for actual and not derived statistics. It is the sum of the (observed minus the expected frequencies) squared divided by the expected frequency. A contingency table is created in the analysis and Yates correction applied if there are only two groups. Fisher's exact test is used if any expected frequency is less than 5. The number of degrees of freedom is the (number of columns -1) multiplied by the (number of rows -1). The value of p is looked up in Chi squared tables based on the number of degrees of freedom.

Ref: Swinscow. Statistics at Square One. BMJ Publications

ANSWER 51

A. FALSE   B. FALSE   C. TRUE   D. FALSE   E. FALSE

Fetal haemoglobin has gamma not delta chains, and is usually 80% replaced by HbA at three months of age, although it can persist through life. It contains the same number of amino-acids as HbA and only weakly binds 2,3 DPG facilitating maternal to foetal oxygen transfer.

Ref: Ganong WF. Review of Medical Physiology. Lange. Ch27.

ANSWER 52

A. TRUE   B. TRUE   C. TRUE   D. TRUE   E. FALSE

Lignocaine hydrochloride is extensively metabolised by hepatic microsomal enzymes such that plasma clearance parallels hepatic blood flow. This accounts for decreased metabolism in low cardiac output states. Of the amide local anaesthetics, prilocaine is metabolised most rapidly.

PHYSICAL:
  Bioavailability 24-46%, pKa 7.7, 64% protein bound

DOSE:

Max 3 mg/kg (7 mg/kg with adrenaline depending on site), toxic over 10 mcg/kg

Ref: Yentis, Hirsch, Smith. Anaesthesia A-Z. Butterworth-Heinemann

ANSWER 53

A. FALSE   B. FALSE   C. FALSE   D. TRUE   E. TRUE

Hypotonic solutions such as dextrose and Hartmann's (osmolarity 272 mOsm/l) worsen cerebral oedema and must be avoided. Steroids, although beneficial in reducing cerebral oedema due to malignancy, have no place in the management of head injury. Lumbar puncture in the presence of elevated ICP may cause coning and is extremely hazardous. Amnesia alone is not an indication for CT.

ANSWER 54

A. FALSE   B. TRUE   C. FALSE   D. FALSE   E. FALSE

Normal pH is associated with a hydrogen ion concentration of 40 nmol/l, maintained principally by the HCO3/CO2 extracellular buffering system. pH is normally measured directly. A normal neonate will initially have an arterial pH of 7.30-7.35.

Ref: Despopoulos A, Silbernagl S. Color Atlas of Physiology. 110-118

ANSWER 55

A. FALSE   B. TRUE   C. FALSE   D. TRUE   E. FALSE

A rise in end tidal carbon dioxide may be due to:

Inspired carbon dioxideRebreathing in the circuit (e.g. disconnection of the inner tube in a Bain circuit or increased dead space)

Increased production of carbon dioxide (e.g. malignant hyperpyrexia)

Inadequate ventilation

Leaks, reduced metabolic rate (due to hypothermia) and impaired cardiac output (pulmonary embolus) all cause reduced end tidal carbon dioxide.

Ref: Dorsch JA, Dorsch SE. Understanding Anesthesia Equipment; Construction, Care and Complications, 2nd edn. Williams & Wilkins, 1984

ANSWER 56

A. FALSE   B. TRUE   C. FALSE   D. TRUE   E. FALSE

It has more affinity for beta receptors: beta:alpha 3:1 following oral ingestion and 7:1 after IV administration. It does have significant ISA and is one of the drugs used in the treatment of the elevated blood pressure of pre-eclampsia.

ANSWER 57

A. FALSE   B. TRUE   C. FALSE   D. FALSE   E. TRUE

Hydrocortisone 10 mg, dexamethasone 750 mcg (0.75 mg). Fludrocortisone is a mineralocorticoid, and doses high enough to have useful glucocorticoid activity would produce unacceptably high degrees of mineralocorticoid activity.

Ref: BNF 1996

ANSWER 58

A. TRUE   B. FALSE   C. FALSE   D. TRUE   E. TRUE

Guillain-Barre occurs 7-10 days after an infectious (usually viral) illness, producing an ascending paralysis. Maximum disability occurs at 4 weeks. Cardiac muscle is involved in muscular dystrophy, and suxamethonium can cause extreme K^+ release. Patients with muscular dystrophy are sensitive to non-depolarising neuromuscular blockers, which must be used with caution in all suspected cases. It is the Eaton-Lambert syndrome which is associated with pulmonary malignancy (specifically with oat cell carcinoma), myasthenia gravis being associated with thymoma in 10% of cases. Eaton-Lambert is a disorder of acetylcholine release, in contrast to myasthenia gravis, which affects the receptor. Muscle function improves with movement, and the Tensilon test (edrophonium) is negative, distinguishing it from myasthenia, where edrophonium relieves the condition for 10 minutes or so and is diagnostic

ANSWER 59

A. TRUE   B. FALSE   C. FALSE   D. TRUE   E. FALSE

Cylinders filled with liquid are marked with a tare weight (empty weight) so the filling can be calculated. In anaesthetic practice we most commonly see the size E cylinder (that can contain 680 litres of oxygen). Carbon dioxide is normally seen in the smaller C size (size F is not made). Entonox has features of both oxygen and nitrous oxide however its filling pressure is similar to that of oxygen (134 bar). Because there is a risk of Entonox separating out into oxygen and nitrous oxide if stored in cold conditions it is recommended that the cylinders are stored lying on their sides to aid re-mixing.

Ref: Dunnill RPH, Colvin MP.   Clinical and Resuscitative Data, 4th edn.   Blackwell Scientific Publications, 1989

ANSWER 60

A. FALSE   B. FALSE   C. TRUE   D. FALSE   E. TRUE

The concept of error and the function of basic measurement display systems is specified in the new Primary syllabus. All systems have a tendency to oscillate at a particular frequency, the resonant frequency. This should be as far removed from the recording frequency and its harmonics as possible and so should be as high as possible. The tendency for machines to over-react to signal changes (over-shoot) is opposed by damping. Critical damping gives no overshoot but a very slow response, so devices should be optimally damped (= 0.64 of critical damping). Pen recorders exhibit errors due to their pivoting motion. This causes arc error and tangential error, not present in oscilloscopic devices. Furthermore pen recorders tend to show hysteresis (a different value produced as the signal is increasing from that produced as the signal is decreasing).

Ref: Sykes MK, Vickers MD, Hull CJ. Principles of Measurement and Monitoring in Anaesthesia and Intensive Care, 3rd edn. Blackwell Scientific Publishers, 1991

ANSWER 61

A. TRUE   B. TRUE   C. TRUE   D. FALSE   E. FALSE

TSH, LH, FSH, and erythropoietin are glycoproteins.

Ref: Despopoulos A, Silbernagl S. Color Atlas of Physiology. 232-271.

ANSWER 62

A. FALSE   **B. FALSE**   **C. FALSE**   **D. TRUE**   **E. TRUE**

Vancomycin is a glycopeptide active against Gram +ve aerobes. Because it is excreted in large amounts in the faeces when given orally it is useful in the treatment of pseudo-membranous colitis. Rapid i.v. infusion can result in drug-induced histamine release and hypotension known as the red man syndrome.

ANSWER 63

A. FALSE   **B. TRUE**   **C. TRUE**   **D. TRUE**   **E. FALSE**

Most organs are under dual control but there are some exceptions. The lacrimal glands are solely parasympathetically innervated. The pupils are dually innervated.

Ref: Yentis, Hirsch, Smith. Anaesthesia A to Z. Butterworth-Heinemann

ANSWER 64

A. TRUE   **B. TRUE**   **C. FALSE**   **D. TRUE**   **E. TRUE**

Local vasodilator metabolites that accumulate in exercise include hydrogen ions, lactic acid and potassium ions but not adenosine. Skeletal muscle arterioles possess sympathetic vasodilator nerves which are cholinergic.

Ref: Ganong WF. Review of Medical Physiology. Lange. Ch31.

ANSWER 65

A. FALSE   **B. TRUE**   **C. FALSE**   **D. FALSE**   **E. TRUE**

Severe cases require intensive care management and frequently require intubation and ventilation. The condition may be insidious in onset, caused by infection, infarction or insufficient insulin. It is characterised by hypovolaemia (osmotic diuresis) and acidosis (ketone body production); large volumes of fluid are needed in resuscitation, but should be dextrose-free until serum glucose has fallen to below 15 mmol/l. There is insulin resistance, and the normal daily requirement will be increased by at least 20%. Insulin therapy causes intracellular uptake of potassium and potassium supplementation is always required. Bicarbonate will only be required in extreme cases with severe systemic acidosis, and rarely with a pH over 7.0. Despite initial high plasma sodium levels, these patients are both salt and water depleted. Initial resuscitation should be with normal saline. Half normal saline may be used with caution.

ANSWER 66

A. TRUE   **B. TRUE**   **C. FALSE**   **D. TRUE**   **E. FALSE**

The placenta plays an important role in hormonal synthesis and secretion, including chorionic gonadotrophin, oestrogens, progesterone, prolactin, somatomammotrophin and renin

Ref: Yentis, Hirsch, Smith. Anaesthesia A to Z. Butterworth-Heinemann.

ANSWER 67

A. FALSE   **B. FALSE**   **C. FALSE**   **D. TRUE**   **E. FALSE**

The technique is an anaesthetic technique and regardless of local practice it should be conducted by suitable qualified anaesthetists with appropriate resuscitation facilities available. Prilocaine 0.5%, without preservative or vasoconstrictor, is the only agent used in contemporary practice, bupivacaine being discarded because of toxicity. The tourniquet should be inflated to twice systolic blood pressure. The quality of postoperative analgesia is disappointing. There is a recognised risk of methaemaglobinaemia with doses of prilocaine in excess of 600 mg.

ANSWER   68
A. FALSE   B. TRUE   C. FALSE   D. TRUE   E. TRUE

Relative humidity is the partial pressure of water vapour divided by the saturated vapour pressure of water at specified temperature, however absolute humidity is the MASS of water vapour in unit volume of air at specified pressure & temperature or the mass concentration (kg/m^3).The Regnault's hygrometer is used to measure RELATIVE humidity and relies in air bubbled through ether that is contained within a silver-coated glass tube. The evaporation of the ether causes a fall in temperature, and the 'dew point' is recorded as the temperature when the relative saturation of the air around the tube becomes 100%. It is marked by water condensing onto the silvered tube. From graphs the relative humidity at the ambient temperature may then be deduced.

Ref: Mushin WM, Jones PL. Physics for the Anaesthetist, 4th edn. Blackwell Scientific Publications, 1987

ANSWER   69
A. FALSE   B. TRUE   C. TRUE   D. FALSE   E. TRUE

Trimetaphan induces hypotension by blocking sympathetic ganglia but it also exhibits some direct vasodilatation. It has a plasma half-life of only 2 minutes. Side-effects include histamine release, mydriasis, and potentiation of succinylcholine, urinary retention and impotence due to the non-selective ganglion blockade.

Ref: Sasada, Smith. Drugs in Anaesthesia & Intensive Care

ANSWER   70
A. TRUE   B. FALSE   C. TRUE   D. FALSE   E. FALSE

Laser is an acronym for Light Amplification by Stimulated Emission of Radiation. It produces light that is powerful because it is parallel, in phase and of specific wavelength. As the light is parallel it does not need focusing, and can be used at varying ranges. However this means that the risks of damage to personnel are still present at long range, and are increased by reflections from shiny surfaces, so matt-surfaced instruments are preferred. The particular lasers used depends on the penetration required. Argon lasers are used on the retina for neo-vascular ablation, carbon dioxide lasers have a penetration of only 200 μm. Medical lasers have many uses including haemostasis, tumour removal and vascular ablation.

Ref: Davis PD, Parbrook GD, Kenny GNC. Basic Physics and Measurement in Anaesthesia, 4th edn. Butterworth-Heinemann, 1995

ANSWER   71
A. FALSE   B. FALSE   C. FALSE   D. FALSE   E. FALSE

It has long been known that electrical equipment could cause death. In America a study on firemen concluded that the danger varied with different AC frequency, and that the highest danger was at 50-60 Hz. Unfortunately another study found that the cheapest frequency was also 50-60 Hz. Economics triumphed over safety!In medical applications the risk of death from ventricular fibrillation is related to the current density at the heart. This means that very small currents (150 μA) may cause VF. It is also possible to get VF in this scenario with low voltages (12 V or less. Equipment for use with patients must conform to BS5724, and equipment with direct cardiac (or major vascular contact) must be of Type CF. This has a maximum 'leakage' current (the danger current) of 50 μA with a single fault. On of the other requirements of BS5724 is that there should NOT be contact between the patient and earth.

Ref: Blunt MC, Urquhart JC. The Anaesthesia Viva: Physics, Measurement, Safety and Clinical Anaesthesia. Greenwich Medical Media, 1996

ANSWER 72

A. FALSE   B. TRUE   C. TRUE   D. FALSE   E. FALSE

Oxytocin is secreted from the posterior pituitary and causes contraction of myoepithelial cells in the walls of the mammary ducts. Uterine sensitivity is enhanced by oestrogen and inhibited by progesterone. Secretion is increased during labour following dilatation of the cervix.

Ref: Ganong WF. Review of Medical Physiology. Lange. Ch14.

ANSWER 73

A. FALSE   B. TRUE   C. TRUE   D. FALSE   E. TRUE

The aortic valve opens early in systole once LV pressure exceeds aortic pressure. It closes at the end of systole. Carotid pressure is highest in mid-systole.

Ref: Ganong WF. Review of Medical Physiology. Lange.

ANSWER 74

A. FALSE   B. TRUE   C. TRUE   D. FALSE   E. TRUE

Hypersensitivity is rare. Long term use carries a risk of osteoporosis.

ANSWER 75

A. TRUE   B. FALSE   C. TRUE   D. TRUE   E. FALSE

Postoperative MI has at least a 50% mortality and occurs most frequently on the third postoperative day; ischaemia is more common at night. The incidence of MI in patients with a recent (less than 3 months) infarct is quoted between 5% and 35%. A DVT may occur in up to 40-80% of those in high risk categories having lower limb surgery, but pulmonary embolism will only happen to a fraction of these and happens after a week, rather than within the first few days.

ANSWER 76

A. FALSE   B. TRUE   C. TRUE   D. FALSE   E. TRUE

Plasma cholinesterase activity may be reduced by:-

Inherited atypical cholinesterase

Acquired deficiency of cholinesterase (hepatic failure, pregnancy, plasmapheresis)

Inhibition of cholinesterase (ecothiopate, cyclophosphamide, phenelzine)

The prolongation of action in genotypically normal patients with acquired deficiencies of the enzyme is usually no longer than 30 minutes. E1u E1u is the commonest genotype and it is present in 96% of the population (DN=75-85 & FN=60); these homozygotes have a completely normal recovery from suxamethonium. In heterozygotes a prolonged action is usually only seen following repeated doses or an infusion. Patients may be heterozygotes for two abnormal brands of plasma cholinesterase. Fluoride resistant enzyme (0.0001% of population) are homozygotes. DN= 65-75 and FN=30.The atypical enzyme (0.03% of population) are homozygotes. DN=15-25 and FN=20. Silent gene (0.001% of population) are homozygotes and have NO cholinesterase activity.

Ref: Watkins J, Levy CJ. Guide to Immediate Anaesthetic Reactions. Butterworth-Heinemann

ANSWER 77

| FALSE | TRUE | FALSE | TRUE | FALSE |

The gold standard for research is the randomised, double blind, controlled trial. Double blinding means neither the patient nor the doctor are aware of the treatment group allocation. Single blinding means the patient is unaware. Ethical committee approval may not be needed for an audit project if there is no departure from accepted clinical practice - auditing admission times to the anaesthetic room, for example. In a research project consent is always needed regardless of the treatment in the control or treatment groups.

ANSWER 78

| A. FALSE | B. TRUE | C. TRUE | D. FALSE | E. FALSE |

TBV=Plasma volume x 100/[100-Hct]. Normal Hct = 47% for males and 42% for females. Blood plasma = 5% body wt; interstitial fluid = 15% body wt; ICF = 40% body wt. In this example, TBV = 5 litres; estimated body weight is 60-65 kg. TBV of 70-75 ml/kg represents a more reasonable estimate in an adult (plasma volume = 3l).

Ref: Ganong WF. Review of Medical Physiology. Lange, Ch 1

ANSWER 79

| A. FALSE | B. FALSE | C. FALSE | D. TRUE | E. TRUE |

Correlation does not indicate causation, merely association. There may or may not be a causative connection between the two variables. The power of a study is 1 minus the beta error (the number of false negatives). The standard error of the mean is the standard deviation divided by the square root of the number in the sample. Transformation can convert a non-normally distributed population into a normal distribution (eg taking the logarithm of the value of a variable).

ANSWER 80

| A. FALSE | B. FALSE | C. FALSE | D. FALSE | E. TRUE |

The P-R interval represents atrial depolarisation and conduction through the AV node, the normal range is 0.12 to 0.2 s. The Q-T interval is normally less than or equal to 0.43 s and the formula for tachycardia is Q-T divided by the square root of the R-R interval.

Ref: Ganong WF. Review of Medical Physiology. Lange.Yentis, Hirsch, Smith. Anaesthesia A toZ. Butterworth-Heinemann.

ANSWER 81

A. FALSE   B. FALSE   C. FALSE   D. FALSE   E. TRUE

Epiglottitis causes a severe systemic upset with fever and drooling, which contrasts with croup where the child may otherwise be well. Croup is seen between six months and three years. Over this age epiglottitis is more likely to be responsible. Cannulation, direct examination and X-rays should not be attempted as laryngospasm may occur. Short term intubation, initially facilitated with sedation but not paralysis, is usually required and the causative organism is Haemophilus; bacterial tracheitis, which is a differential diagnosis, is caused by Staphylococcus.

Ref: Johnston D, Hull D. Essential Paediatrics, 3rd edn. Churchill Livingstone, 1994

ANSWER 82

A. TRUE   B. TRUE   C. FALSE   D. FALSE   E. TRUE

Base excess is used to assess the metabolic component of the blood-gas analysis. it is defined as the amount of strong acid that must be added to 1 litre of the blood to produce a pH of 7.40 at a pCO_2 of 5.3 kPa and 37°C. Oxygen content measurement requires a co-oximeter and is not available from the normal blood gas analyser. Errors can occur due to excessive heparin either due to the dilutional effect of excessive saline (low pCO_2 and low pO_2, though the pH is little effected), or due to the heparin itself (high potassium measurement). Prolonged storage even at 4°C can lead to either a falsely low reading of pO2 (due to ongoing metabolism in white blood cells) or a falsely high reading (due to bubbles dissolving).

Ref: Dorsch JA, Dorsch SE. Understanding Anesthesia Equipment; Construction, Care and Complications, 2nd edn. Williams & Wilkins, 1984

ANSWER 83

A. TRUE   B. TRUE   C. FALSE   D. TRUE   E. FALSE

Sine waves are defined by their wavelength, amplitude and phase. They are the building blocks for all waveforms, as complex waves can all be broken down into sine waves (Fourier analysis). The addition of two waves of equal frequency depends on their phase shift, and two waves exactly 180° out of phase will cancel each other out. All electromagnetic waves travel at 3×10^8 m/s including radio waves, infra-red, visible and ultraviolet light as well as X-rays. EEG waves are divided into four groups according to frequency (ordered delta, theta, alpha and beta from lowest to highest).

Ref: Davis PD, Parbrook GD, Kenny GNC. Basic Physics and Measurement in Anaesthesia, 4th edn. Butterworth-Heinemann, 1995

ANSWER 84

A. TRUE   B. TRUE   C. FALSE   D. FALSE   E. TRUE

Mass spectrometry and Raman scattering are the only methods presently available that allow the machine to identify the gas present, however light absorption (both infra-red and ultra-violet) allow determination of the concentration of a known gas. Thermal conductivity is used (rarely) to measure inorganic gases and paramagnetism for oxygen measurement.

Ref: Sykes MK, Vickers MD, Hull, CJ. Principles of Measurement and Monitoring in Anaesthesia and Intensive Care, 3rd edn. Blackwell Scientific Publishers, 1991

ANSWER 85

A. FALSE   B. TRUE   C. TRUE   D. FALSE   E. TRUE

The risk of coronary steal from isoflurane preferentially dilating healthy coronary vessels at the expense of diseased ones has been postulated but never proven. Hypertension is associated with subendocardial ischaemia due to left ventricular hypertrophy. Any patient who has had an infarct is at higher risk of a peroperative reinfarction than the general population. The risk is inversely related to the interval from infarct to anaesthesia, and greatest within the first three months where it ranges from 5 to 35 % with a very high mortality.

ANSWER 86

A. FALSE   B. TRUE   C. TRUE   D. TRUE   E. TRUE

Solutions of barbiturates are stable at room temperature for up to two weeks; however as they contain no antibacterial agents should only be used if made up less than 24 hours previously. Hepatic clearance of methohexitone is about three times greater than thiopentone. It is about 2.5 times as potent as thiopentone. Barbiturates decrease cerebral blood flow, intracranial pressure and cerebral oxygen requirements.

PHYSICAL:

pH 11, pKa 7.9, 55% albumin bound

DOSE:

1.0-1.5 mg/kg.

Ref: Nimmo, Rowbotham, Smith. Anaesthesia, Blackwell

ANSWER 87

A. TRUE   B. FALSE   C. FALSE   D. TRUE   E. TRUE

Sevoflurane is indeed a hexafluoroisopropyl fluromethyl ether. It is related to isoflurane, enflurance and desflurane which are all also ethers. Halothane is a hydrocarbon. About 5% undergoes biotransformation in the liver. It does not possess a -CF2H group and thus produces no CO when in contact with very dry sodalime (this property is shared with halothane). Its SVP at 20 degrees C is 160 mmHg (isoflurane 238 mmHg), its BP is 56 degrees C (isoflurane 48.5, enflurane 56.5) and its blood:gas partition coefficient is 0.69 (isoflurane 1.15).

Ref: British Journal of Anaesthesia 1996; 76: 435-445 (excellent review article)

ANSWER 88

A. TRUE   B. FALSE   C. TRUE   D. TRUE   E. TRUE

Diathermy must be used with caution as it may deprogramme a pacemaker or induce a current in the wire, injuring the myocardium. The fasciculations associated with suxamethonium may cause inhibition of pacing. The coding refers to the chamber paced, the chamber sensed, and the response. The indications for pacing are complete heart block, symptomatic heart block, trifascicular block and the sick sinus syndrome.

Ref: Juste et al. Minimising cardiac risk. Anaesthesia 1996;51:255

ANSWER   89

A. TRUE   B. TRUE   C. FALSE   D. FALSE   E. TRUE

Standard deviation is the square root of the variance. The standard error of the mean is the standard deviation divided by the square root of the number observed.

ANSWER   90

A. FALSE   B. TRUE   C. TRUE   D. TRUE   E. TRUE

A single breath technique using pure oxygen may be used to estimate anatomical dead space, closing volume, and residual volume based on dynamic changes in the expired nitrogen concentration. The Bohr equation measures physiolgical dead space vs alveolar volume based on fractional concentrations of expired, inspired and alveolar CO_2.

Ref: Ganong WF. Review of Medical Physiology. Lange, Ch34

Exam 4

QUESTION 1

In a normally distributed population

A. Over 50% of the individuals are normal
B. 15% of the observations will be outside of 2 standard deviations from the mean
C. As many values are above the mean as below it
D. The variance is twice the standard deviation
E. The variance is a function of the mean

QUESTION 2

Congenital heart lesions

A. Murmurs are invariably associated with valvular defects
B. A heart lesion is detected in 70 per 1,000 live births
C. Coarctation of the aorta is a cyanotic lesion
D. Beta-blockade is useful in the management of the cardiac failure associated with certain cyanotic cardiac lesions
E. The Eisenmenger syndrome involves a left-to-right shunt

QUESTION 3

Anaesthetic breathing circuits

A. Lack and Bain circuits have similar flow characteristics
B. A Mapleson E circuit is efficient for spontaneously breathing patients
C. A Jackson-Rees modified circuit has a valve with a release pressure of 2 cmH_2O
D. A coaxial Lack circuit has the expired gas passing in the outer tubing
E. The tubing is corrugated to improve flow characteristics

QUESTION 4

Regarding probability

A. A p value of $p<0.05$ is taken as significant when considering biological systems
B. A p value of $p<0.05$ means that if the test were repeated 20 times, it would produce a significant result once by chance alone
C. A p value of $p<0.05$ implies clinical significance
D. A value for p can be obtained from descriptive statistics
E. Probability is expressed as p

QUESTION 5

Concerning errors in statistics

A. The power of a study describes the likelihood of detecting a real difference if it exists
B. A type 1 error is the same as the alpha-error
C. A type 1 error is a false negative
D. The commonest cause of a type 2 error is that the sample size was too small
E. A type 1 error is unlikely to influence the conclusions of a trial

QUESTION 6

Concerning pain pathways

A. A-delta and C fibres have cell bodies within the dorsal root ganglion of the spinal cord
B. A-delta fibres synapse with cells of the substantia gelatinosa of the spinal cord
C. C fibres synapse with cells in laminae II and III in the dorsal horn
D. Most ascending neurones are in the anterolateral columns
E. The substantia gelatinosa does not project directly to higher levels

QUESTION 7

Prolonged positive pressure ventilation (IPPV) is associated with

A. Surgical emphysema
B. Acalculous cholecystitis
C. Reduction in pulmonary compliance
D. Tracheal stenosis
E. Increased extravascular fluid

QUESTION 8

Phenoxybenzamine

A. Is a non-selective alpha-adrenergic antagonist
B. Acts predominantly on post-synaptic alpha-1 receptors
C. Causes mydriasis
D. May result in nasal stuffiness
E. Is useful in the management of craniopharyngioma

QUESTION 9

The following promote intracellular uptake of potassium

A. Aldosterone
B. Adrenaline
C. Acidosis
D. Insulin
E. 2,3-DPG

QUESTION 10

When measuring glomerular filtration rate

A. Renal blood flow must be measured or estimated
B. An indicator substance must not undergo reabsorption following tubular excretion
C. The result matches clearance of the indicator if it is renally inert
D. One would expect approximately 180 litres to be filtered daily
E. Use of sodium as an indicator would lead to an erroneously high GFR

QUESTION 11

The following increase pulmonary vascular resistance

A. Maximal inspiration
B. Anaemia
C. Maximal expiration
D. Histamine
E. Prostacyclin

QUESTION 12

In emergency obstetric anaesthesia for Caesarean section, the following are definite indications for general anaesthesia

A. Fetal bradycardia
B. Antepartum haemorrhage
C. Maternal dissatisfaction with regional blockade
D. Obstetric request
E. Platelet count below 80,000/ml

QUESTION 13

Concerning fluid therapy

A. Oliguria can be reliably managed with a loop diuretic
B. Artificial colloids should be used in preference to natural colloids for volume replacement
C. There is no risk of infection with natural colloids
D. Hydroxyethyl starch (HES) prolongs partial thromboplastin time
E. The volume of colloid required in the management of acute anaphylaxis is 10 ml/kg

QUESTION 14

Biological signals

A. Signal voltage from an EEG is much larger than that from an EMG
B. Auditory evoked potentials are measured by summation of many individual signals
C. An ECG electrode contains aluminium as its basis
D. Amplifiers used in displaying the ECG rely on common mode rejection to improve the signal to noise ratio
E. The P wave of the ECG is normally positive in all leads because it is a depolarisation wave

QUESTION   15

The ileum is the main site of absorption of

A. Iron
B. B_{12}
C. Glucose
D. Bile salts
E. Fat soluble vitamins

QUESTION   16

Smooth muscle

A. Has a longer action potential than cardiac muscle
B. Can be tetanized
C. Is a syncytium
D. Has pacemaker cells
E. Has no sarcomeres

QUESTION   17

The following types of lasers are used in medicine

A. Helium
B. Carbon dioxide
C. Argon
D. Sodium
E. Neodymium-YAG (yttrium aluminium garnet)

QUESTION   18

Dipalmitoylphosphatidylcholine

A. Is a mucopolypeptide
B. Causes a decrease in surface tension
C. Causes an increase in chest wall compliance
D. Production is reduced after prolonged reduction in pulmonary blood flow
E. Maintains the same surface tension for different sized alveoli

QUESTION   19

Ephedrine

A. Contains a catechol ring
B. Causes the stimulation of both alpha and beta adrenoceptors
C. Owes all of its action to the effects of the release of noradrenaline.
D. Increases uterine tone
E. Can exist in four isomeric forms, two of which are pharmacologically active.

QUESTION 20

Warfarin activity is affected by the following interactions

A. Rifampicin decreases its effect by inducing hepatic microsomal enzymes
B. Cimetidine enhances its effect by decreasing the rate of warfarin metabolism
C. Chloral hydrate enhances its effect by displacing warfarin from albumin binding sites
D. Allopurinol decreases its effect by altering the hepatic receptor site for the drug
E. Barbiturates decrease its effect by enhancing the synthesis of clotting factors

QUESTION 21

Distortion of the trace seen in direct arterial monitoring is increased by

A. Bubbles
B. Connections in the tubing
C. Shortening the tubing
D. Increasing the diameter of the tubing
E. Clots in the cannula

QUESTION 22

In the rapid sequence induction

A. Cricoid pressure is applied with a force of 40 Newtons
B. Cricoid pressure must never be released until the tracheal tube is correctly located and the cuff inflated
C. Misting in the catheter mount is a reliable indicator of correct placement of the tracheal tube
D. The lungs should be manually inflated with 100% oxygen until intubation is achieved
E. Pretreatment with alfentanil is used to reduce the pressor response to intubation

QUESTION 23

Central venous pressure (CVP) measurements

A. +5 mmHg is higher than +5 cmH$_2$O
B. CVP is a reliable indicator of left ventricular performance
C. The catheter should be placed in the right atrium
D. A normal CVP excludes a diagnosis of pulmonary oedema
E. The value of CVP is unaffected by therapeutic vasoconstriction

QUESTION 24

Vagal efferent stimulation causes

A. Increased insulin secretion
B. Decreased physiological dead space
C. Decreased gastrin secretion
D. Increased gastric acid secretion
E. Reduced bile production

QUESTION   25

Hyoscine

A. Is a less potent anti-sialagogue than atropine
B. Does not cross the blood-brain barrier
C. Is largely excreted unchanged in the urine
D. Can be used in the treatment of motion sickness
E. May produce excitement and restlessness

QUESTION   26

The following cause a fall in the measured end-tidal carbon dioxide level (assuming constant spontaneous ventilation)

A. Endobroncheal intubation
B. Failure of the nitrous oxide supply in a patient breathing 66% N_2O through a Bain circuit
C. Shivering
D. Cardiac arrest
E. Extreme hypoventilation

QUESTION   27

In laminar flow through a tube

A. Flow is proportional to viscosity of the fluid
B. Flow is proportional to the pressure gradient
C. Flow is inversely proportional to density
D. Flow is proportional to the forth power of radius
E. Flow nearest the wall of the tube will be almost zero

QUESTION   28

Peripheral chemoreceptors

A. Are found in the carotid sinus
B. Give rise to increased afferent signals when PaO_2 falls below 13 kPa
C. Are downregulated in the presence of chronic lung disease
D. Maintain $PaCO_2$ within the range 4.5-6.0 kPa
E. Are stimulated by elevated levels of carboxyhaemoglobin

QUESTION   29

Alpha-1 adrenergic receptor stimulation leads to

A. Increased lipolysis
B. Glycogenolysis in the liver
C. Gut relaxation
D. Increased release of insulin
E. Bronchodilation

QUESTION 30

Pulmonary blood flow

- A. Is normally less than the cardiac output
- B. Has a mean arterial pressure of 2 kPa
- C. In zone 1 occurs mainly during diastole
- D. Of 5000 ml/min with a minute ventilation of 7 litres suggests the presence of a shunt
- E. Is maximal in zone 2

QUESTION 31

The Tec 4 vaporiser

- A. Has a cloth wick to aid complete vaporisation
- B. Has a Selectatec mount that stops its concomitant use with another Selectatec vaporiser
- C. Under COSHH regulations should be refilled in a fume cupboard
- D. Has a bimetallic strip to provide temperature compensation
- E. Has a system to reduce the risk of filling with the incorrect agent

QUESTION 32

Remifentanil

- A. Is a derivative of fentanyl with an ether linkage
- B. Has a speed of onset similar to fentanyl
- C. Can be administered safely by the spinal or epidural route
- D. Is dependent on pseudo-cholinesterase for its breakdown
- E. Should be avoided in renal failure

QUESTION 33

Muscle spindles

- A. Consist of a single encapsulated extrafusal muscle fibre
- B. Have their own motor nerve supply
- C. Maintain muscle length by initiation of the stretch reflex
- D. Reduce the magnitude of physiological tremor
- E. Convey impulses via A-beta fibres to the spinal cord

QUESTION 34

A man with blood group B+

- A. Can only have children of blood group O or B
- B. His father was possibly blood group O+
- C. If the mother of his children is blood group B+ the children can only be blood group B+
- D. Has the rarest blood group
- E. Can be safely transfused with group O+ blood in an emergency

QUESTION 35

The following have anti-emetic activity

A. Chlorpromazine
B. Hyoscine
C. Chlormethiazole
D. Moclobemide
E. Phenytoin

QUESTION 36

Cardiac output can be measured using

A. CO_2 and mass spectrometry
B. Impedance plethysmography
C. Electromagnetic flow measurement
D. Ballistocardiography
E. Aortovelography

QUESTION 37

Thyroid hormones

A. Increase oxygen consumption in the anterior pituitary
B. Increase the absorption of carbohydrate from the intestine
C. Cause a fall in red cell 2,3–DPG levels
D. Indirectly cause an increase in nitrogen excretion in adults
E. Inhibit cardiac muscle adenylate cyclase

QUESTION 38

Aldosterone

A. Stimulates mRNA synthesis
B. Increases Na reabsorption from saliva
C. Excess results in hypotension
D. Is secreted from the juxta glomerular cells
E. Release is stimulated by a rise in angiotensin II

QUESTION 39

Organophosphorus compounds

A. Are readily absorbed across the skin
B. Inhibit acetylcholinesterase by phosphorylation of the anionic site of the enzyme
C. Are often also inhibitors of plasma cholinesterase
D. Can cause autonomic instability
E. Can have their action reversed by pralidoxime, which reactivates acetyl-cholinesterase

QUESTION 40

Mannitol

A. Is readily absorbed from the gastrointestinal tract
B. Is a six carbon sugar
C. Enters cells by an active transport mechanism
D. Is completely filtered at the renal glomeruli, with none of the drug subsequently reabsorbed from the renal tubule
E. Increases urinary excretion of water, sodium, chloride and bicarbonate

QUESTION 41

Prostacyclin (Epoprostenol, Flolan)

A. Is indicated as an alternative to heparin during renal dialysis
B. Is a weak inhibitor of platelet aggregation
C. May produce hypotension
D. Is presented as a freeze dried preparation of the sodium salt
E. Inhibits platelet aggregation at a dose of approximately 5 mcg/kg/min

QUESTION 42

A two compartment model

A. Implies entero-hepatic recirculation
B. Is characterized by an exponential plasma decay curve
C. Indicates both hepatic and renal metabolism are occurring
D. Requires the application of two rate constants
E. Is used to construct a control group during drug trials

QUESTION 43

Salmeterol

A. Is similar in structure to salbutamol
B. Is equally as potent at the beta-1 and beta-2 adrenoceptor
C. Is short-acting
D. Is useful in the treatment of an acute asthmatic attack
E. Tachyphylaxis to bronchodilator properties is common

QUESTION 44

Propofol

A. Is associated with dystonic type reactions in some patients
B. Is highly protein bound in plasma
C. Is presented as an emulsion containing soyabean oil, glycerol, egg phosphatide, sodium hydroxide and water
D. Is metabolised predominantly in the liver to inactive metabolites and a corresponding quinol
E. Can safely be used in both malignant hyperpyrexia and porphyria

QUESTION 45

Midazolam

A. Is active in its water soluble form
B. Is more lipophilic than the other benzodiazepines
C. Is extensively protein bound
D. Accumulates significantly in oliguric renal failure
E. Has a bimodally distributed elimination half life with about 6% having a half life of greater than 8 hours

QUESTION 46

Sinus arrhythmia

A. Occurs in the elderly
B. Is rarely present in athletes
C. Causes an increased R-R interval during inspiration
D. Involves the stellate ganglion
E. Is more marked on exertion

QUESTION 47

The standard error of the mean

A. Equals the square root of the standard deviation divided by the number in the sample
B. Is related to the variance of the population
C. Is large when the number in the sample is small
D. May be used to calculate the likelihood that two samples come from the same population
E. Estimates the standard deviation of the means of samples taken from the same population

QUESTION 48

Deposition of new bone

A. Is stimulated by calcitonin
B. Is stimulated by a high local phosphate concentration
C. Is dependent upon alkaline phosphatase activity
D. Occurs as a result of osteoclast activation
E. Occurs when the solubility product of calcium and phosphate is exceeded

QUESTION 49

Thiopentone

A. Is a powder which is made up with normal saline
B. Is stored with sodium hydroxide to alkalinise it
C. In solution has a pH of 10.8
D. Has an elimination half life of 65 minutes
E. May cause a tachycardia due to a direct effect on beta-1 receptors in the heart

QUESTION 50

Milrinone

A. Is one of the imidazolone derivative group of phosphodiesterase inhibitors.
B. Is structurally related to amrinone
C. Has a short (10-20 minutes) terminal half life making it well suited to use as an infusion
D. Is excreted largely unchanged by the kidneys
E. Is incompatible with intravenous frusemide when given through the same cannula

QUESTION 51

Enflurane

A. Is more potent than isoflurane
B. Is the volatile agent of first choice for patients with renal impairment
C. Is a halogenated ether
D. Causes less respiratory depression than halothane
E. Has an SVP lower than that of halothane

QUESTION 52

The following drugs relax uterine smooth muscle

A. Propofol
B. Isoflurane
C. Ritodrine
D. Magnesium
E. Salbutamol

QUESTION 53

Regarding the Stellate ganglion block

A. Chassaignac's tubercle represents the bony landmark
B. It is performed for anaesthesia of the upper limb
C. A Horner's syndrome is unlikely
D. Complications include a subarachnoid block
E. Pneumothorax is unlikely

QUESTION 54

Concerning the carotid body

A. Its oxygen demands are met largely by dissolved oxygen
B. It receives less blood per ml of tissue than brain
C. It is more responsive to changes in oxygen tension than oxygen content
D. Its discharge is not increased in carbon monoxide toxicity
E. Its discharge is increased by a fall in mean arterial blood pressure

QUESTION 55

In the fetal circulation at birth

A. The pulmonary vascular resistance halves
B. Left atrial pressure falls
C. The foramen ovale fuses
D. The umbilical veins constrict
E. The fetus receives a placental transfusion

QUESTION 56

Concerning sevoflurane

A. It is a poly-fluorinated ether
B. Less than 1% is metabolised
C. It is a suitable induction agent for children
D. It has physical properties resembling desflurane
E. It is not degraded by soda-lime

QUESTION 57

Syntocinon

A. Has a weak antidiuretic effect
B. May cause palpitations if given rapidly intravenously
C. Commonly causes hypertension
D. Causes umbilical artery vasodilation
E. Mediates uterine smooth muscle contraction independent of the level of circulating oestrogens

QUESTION 58

Iron

A. About 15% of ingested iron is absorbed
B. Most of dietary iron is in the ferrous state
C. Iron is best absorbed in the ferric state
D. Iron is not absorbed in the stomach
E. Pancreatic juice inhibits iron absorption

QUESTION 59

The following drugs have been reported to be teratogenic

A. Carbamezepine
B. Nitrous oxide
C. Warfarin
D. Phenytoin
E. Sodium valproate

QUESTION 60

A mole

A. Is a basic SI unit
B. Of any liquid will have the same volume
C. Of diamond weighs approximately 12 grams
D. Of oxygen will occupy 22.4 litres at standard temperature and pressure
E. Will contain Newton's number of particles

QUESTION 61

In suxamethonium apnoea

A. Muscle biopsy is included in the postoperative investigation
B. Once identified, the patient with the condition must be sedated and ventilated until neuromuscular function returns
C. Transfusion of fresh frozen plasma should be used
D. The condition is inherited in an autosomal dominant fashion
E. Enhancement of dibucaine inhibition indicates the presence of the condition

QUESTION 62

The following may precipitate an episode of acute intermittent porphyria

A. Methohexitone
B. Pethidine
C. Droperidol
D. Phenytoin
E. Tolbutamide

QUESTION 63

With regard to anti-emetics

A. Metoclopramide has a central and a peripheral effect
B. Phenothiazines are anti-emetics because they are agonists at dopamine receptors in the CNS
C. Droperidol can cause sedation, restlessness, anxiety and dystonia
D. Cyclizine is an anti-histamine and has a high incidence of extrapyramidal side effects
E. Ondansetron has a plasma half-life of about 6 hours

QUESTION 64

The Goldman Cardiac Risk Index

A. The presence of angina indicates high risk with a score of 8 points
B Predicts postoperative outcome
C. Is used to identify patients at risk of major perioperative cardiac complications
D. The highest risk applies to patients with cardiac failure
E. Is a highly sensitive but poorly specific index

QUESTION 65

During a valsalva

A. An initial reduction in blood pressure on glottic opening is normal
B. Prolonged reduction in blood pressure during glottic closure may represent autonomic dysfunction
C. Bradycardia on glottic opening is abnormal
D. Tachycardia during glottic closure is normal
E. A decrease in middle ear pressure occurs

QUESTION 66

Bronchial asthma

A. Medical treatment includes ipratropium, salbutamol, steroids, aminophylline, ephedrine and cromoglycate
B. Pulsus paradoxus is a deficit in the pulse rate between inspiration and expiration
C. Hypokalaemia is a complication of therapy
D. Chest X-ray is an essential preoperative investigation
E. Arterial blood gas analysis should be performed prior to elective surgery

QUESTION 67

The following drugs cause prolongation of the Q-T interval

A. Sotalol
B. Quinidine
C. Verapamil
D. Flecainide
E. Disopyramide

QUESTION 68

Heparin

A. Has the same mode of action as the low molecular weight heparins (LMWH)
B. Relies for its action on an adequate concentration of antithrombin III
C. Has a longer duration of action than the LMWH
D. Binds to antithrombin III and thrombin
E. May have its anticoagulant effects reversed by the administration of protamine at a dose of 1 mg protamine to every 100 mg of heparin

QUESTION 69

Infra-red absorption spectrometry

A. Is only useful as a capnometer in research applications
B. Relies on Beer's Law
C. The sample chamber has sapphire windows because these filter the incident light
D. Carbon dioxide absorption is measured at 4.3 μm
E. Has a response time of faster than 100 msec

QUESTION 70

Calculation of Nernst's equation

A. Requires knowledge of the gas constant
B. Requires knowledge of the Faraday constant
C. Enables estimation of intracellular ionic concentrations
D. For potassium in the resting motor neurone = -70 mV
E. Will return a negative potential if intracellular concentration is greater than extracellular concentration

QUESTION 71

Scavenging systems

A. Should provide a negative pressure of at least 2 cmH_2O
B. Should discharge outside away from working areas
C. Are required under UK law
D. Are connected to the anaesthetic circuit with a 22 mm connector
E. Activated charcoal successfully absorbs volatile anaesthetic agents

QUESTION 72

Respiratory compliance

A. Lung compliance is less than total thoracic compliance
B. Static compliance can be measured with a spirometer and a simple water manometer
C. In IPPV, tidal volume depends only on lung compliance
D. Dynamic compliance is measured when gas is being expired
E. Is related to body size

QUESTION 73

The following statements about the synthetic gelatins are true

A. They have an average molecular weight of 70 000 daltons
B. Succinylated gelatins are associated with potentially severe allergic reactions
C. Prior exposure is necessary for severe anaphylaxis
D. There is an increased risk of pulmonary oedema associated with their use compared to the modified starch preparations
E. The risk of anaphylactoid reactions is increased in non-anaesthetised normovolaemic patients

QUESTION 74

Concerning synaptic transmission

A. The synaptic cleft is 30 μm wide
B. Temporal summation may occur
C. Synaptic delay is normally 0.5 ms
D. IPSP's are depolarising
E. EPSP's are hyperpolarising

QUESTION 75

In pregnancy

A. Red cell mass expansion exceeds plasma expansion
B. The blood becomes hypocoagulable
C. Factor VII levels increase
D. Fibrin degradation products increase
E. Platelet count decreases

QUESTION 76

In statistical analysis

A. A value p<0.001 indicates great significance
B. The Chi-squared test may be used with ordinal data
C. Student's t-test may be used to compare pairs of data from the same subjects
D. A parameter may be a measurement or an outcome
E. A population is a group of subjects with no common feature

QUESTION 77

Anaesthesia at high altitude (using a plenum vaporiser)

A. The concentration delivered by the vaporiser will be higher than the dialled value
B. The concentration dialled into the vaporiser will need to be higher for the same effect
C. The concentration dialled into the vaporiser will need to be lower for the same effect
D. The inspired oxygen concentration may need to be increased
E. The anaesthetic potency of 50% nitrous oxide will be reduced

QUESTION 78

The volume of distribution of a drug is determined by

A. The pKa
B. The extent of plasma protein binding
C. The extent of tissue binding
D. The rate of excretion
E. The total aqueous volume available

QUESTION 79

Pulse oximetry

A. Tricuspid incompetence leads to a falsely low reading
B. The pulse oximeter is designed to measure the light absorption every 0.5 sec
C. A rapid response to changes in alveolar gas tensions can be expected
D. The light for measurement comes from a filtered light source
E. Carboxyhaemoglobin concentration in heavy smokers may lead to a reading that is falsely high by 10-15%

QUESTION 80

The Basic SI units include

A. The metre
B. The second
C. The volt
D. The gram
E. The curie

QUESTION 81

During the cardiac cycle

A. Mitral valve closure immediately precedes the JVP c wave
B. The T wave of the ECG is seen just before the mitral valve opens
C. Isovolumetric contraction precedes the 1st heart sound
D. An ejection fraction of >80% is considered normal
E. Duration of systole shortens when the heart rate increases

QUESTION 82

When setting up a ventilator to provide intermittent positive pressure ventilation in theatre

A. If a circle system is in use the fresh gas flow must not exceed 3 l/min
B. The tidal volume may be calculated as 7-10 ml/kg in the adult
C. When using a minute volume divider the fresh gas flow should exceed the required minute volume by 10%
D. When using the Penlon Nuffield with a Bain attachment the APL valve must be tightly closed
E. End-tidal carbon dioxide provides an accurate indication of the adequacy of ventilation

QUESTION 83

Monitoring neuromuscular blockade

A. The stimulator should deliver a current of 60-70 mA
B. There should be no fade with a 5 second tetanic stimulus in an unparalysed patient
C. Fade is a feature of depolarising blockade
D. Head lift is a poor indicator of post-operative recovery of neuromuscular function
E. Persisting suxamethonium blockade can be excluded if the train-of-four pattern shows fade

QUESTION 84

The following drugs may safely be given to patients with hepatic porphyria

A. Pethidine
B. Thiopentone
C. Phenytoin
D. Warfarin
E. Diazepam

QUESTION 85

Neutrophilia (>7000/microlitre) can occur in association with

A. Pregnancy
B. Trauma
C. Viral infection
D. Steroid therapy
E. Acute haemorrhage

QUESTION 86

Concerning the blood supply to the placenta

A. Maternal placental blood flow is about 400 ml/min at term
B. Umbilical blood flow is approximately 300 ml/min at term
C. Umbilical arterial PO_2 is greater than umbilical venous PO_2
D. Normally there are two umbilical veins
E. Maternal placental blood flow is inversely related to uterine vascular resistance

QUESTION 87

Hydralazine

A. Dilates arterioles and veins equally
B. Undergoes extensive first pass metabolism, the degree of which depends on the acetylator status of the patient
C. Increases heart rate, stroke volume and cardiac output
D. May cause a lupus-like syndrome after a single dose
E. Decreases renin activity

QUESTION 88

Erythromycin

A. Can be bactericidal or bacteriostatic against Gram positive anaerobes
B. When given intravenously may result in thrombophlebitis
C. Inhibits protein synthesis by bacteria ribosomes
D. Increases gut transit time
E. May potentiate the effects of warfarin.

QUESTION 89

A drug that is 98% protein bound

A. Will double its free drug concentration if protein binding is decreased to 96%
B. Will show a 2% increase in free drug concentration if protein binding falls 2%
C. Must have a pKa > 7.4
D. Might be diazepam
E. Might be midazolam

QUESTION 90

A body plethysmograph can be used to measure

A. Compliance
B. Work of breathing
C. Gas exchange
D. Airway resistance
E. FEV_1

Exam 4: Answers

ANSWER 1

A. FALSE   B. FALSE   C. TRUE   D. FALSE   E. FALSE

In a normally distributed population, mean, median and mode have the same value. The variance is the square of the standard deviation. The standard deviation is the square root of the sum of the squares of (x - mean of x) divided by number of observations - 1.

+/-1 SD includes 68% of the population.

+/-2 SD 96%.

+/-3 SD 99.7%

ANSWER 2

A. FALSE   B. FALSE   C. FALSE   D. TRUE   E. FALSE

The Eisenmenger syndrome describes a left-to-right shunt reversing and becoming right-to-left. Irreversible pulmonary hypertension arises as a consequence. Deoxygenated blood enters the systemic circulation and cyanosis is evident. Innocent systolic murmurs may be heard in 72% of schoolchildren, but a lesion is present in only 7 per 1,000 live births. Murmurs may be due to septal defects or to coarctation and are not invariably associated with a valvular lesion. Beta-blockade is used to relieve infundibular spasm in Fallot's tetralogy.

Ref: The preoperative management of the child with a heart murmur. Paediatric Anaesthesia 1995; 5: 151-156

ANSWER 3

A. FALSE   B. FALSE   C. FALSE   D. FALSE   E. FALSE

Mapleson's classification of breathing systems is a basic part of the learning of trainee anaesthetists. The Lack circuit is a modification of the Magill attachment, and is Mapleson A, efficient for spontaneous ventilation. It has the fresh gas flow passing in the outer tubing and the expiratory gases into the inner limb. The Bain circuit is Mapleson D and is more efficient for controlled ventilation, as is the Jackson-Rees modification (Mapleson F). The latter consists of a bag on the expiratory limb of the circuit, with no valve. This minimises resistance and so is ideal for paediatric anaesthesia. The tubing is corrugated to reduce the risk of kinking and corrugation will worsen flow characteristics by promoting turbulence.

Ref: Davis PD, Parbrook GD, Kenny GNC. Basic Physics and Measurement in Anaesthesia, 4th edn. Butterworth-Heinemann, 1995

ANSWER 4

A. TRUE   B. TRUE   C. FALSE   D. FALSE   E. TRUE

Clinical significance can never be assumed from statistical significance, however well-designed the trial. A value for p can only be derived from inferential statistical methods; descriptive methods only identify the presence or otherwise of a central tendency in data, and generate means, medians and modes.

ANSWER 5

A. TRUE   B. TRUE   C. FALSE   D. TRUE   E. FALSE

A type 1 error (which is the same as the alpha error) is a false positive. The commonest reason for a type 1 error is multiple testing. A type 2 error (beta error) is a false negative, and is likely to have happened because the sample size - the number studied - was too small. The power of a study describes the likelihood of detecting a real difference if it exists and is =[(1-type 2 error) x 100%]. Power analysis should be performed prior to a clinical trial to determine the numbers required in the study groups to show a specified difference (which is selected on the basis of a required clinically significant difference). It may also be applied retrospectively when assessing the validity of a statistically insignificant result.

Ref: Yentis, Hirsch, Smith. Anaesthesia A to Z. Butterworth-Heinemann

ANSWER 6

A. TRUE   B. FALSE   C. TRUE   D. TRUE   E. TRUE

First order neurones (A-delta and C) have cell bodies within the dorsal root ganglia, A-delta fibres synapse with cells in laminae I and V of the dorsal horn whereas C fibres synapse with cells in the substantia gelatinosa (laminae II and III). The SG does not project directly to higher levels but contains multiple interneurones involved in pain modification. Most second order neurones cross within a few segments and ascend in the anterolateral columns (spinothalamic tract).

Ref: Yentis, Hirsch, Smith. Anaesthesia A to Z. Butterworth-Heinemann

ANSWER 7

A. TRUE   B. TRUE   C. TRUE   D. TRUE   E. TRUE

Surgical emphysema is a consequence of intubation, barotrauma, positive pressure and pneumothorax. Cholestasis and acalculous cholecystitis occur in long-term ventilated intensive care patients. Pulmonary fluid retention, fibrosis and tracheal stenosis (with post-extubation stridor) are common consequences. IPPV has an anti-diuretic effect and interstitial oedema is common.

ANSWER 8

A. TRUE   B. TRUE   C. FALSE   D. TRUE   E. FALSE

Phenoxybenzamine is a non-selective alpha blocker. Blockade is competitive but non reversible. It causes miosis commonly and not mydriasis. It leads to a decrease in systemic vascular resistance, decreased diastolic blood pressure and marked orthostatic hypotension. It is used in the treatment of phaeochromocytomas to reduce the alpha effects of uncontrolled adrenaline release in the preoperative phase. It has a long half life when given both orally and intravenously.

Ref: Sasada, Smith. Drugs in Anaesthesia & Intensive Care.

ANSWER 9

A. TRUE   B. TRUE   C. FALSE   D. TRUE   E. FALSE

Acute regulation of extracellular K concentration is achieved by redistribution. Normally 98-99% resides intracellularly. Movement is controlled largely by release of insulin in the presence of hyperkalaemia, and the effects of alkalosis, adrenaline and aldosterone release. Chronic regulation is primarily achieved by the kidney and colon.

Ref: Despopoulos A, Silbernagl S. Color Atlas of Physiology, 120-152

ANSWER 10

A. FALSE   B. FALSE   C. TRUE   D. TRUE   E. FALSE

GFR measurements are made using renally inert indicators where passive rate of filtration at the glomerulus = rate of excretion. GFR x Plasma conc. = Urine flow rate x Urine conc. Renal blood flow will alter GFR but does not need to be measured. Na reabsorption leads to a low excretion rate and low urine concentration.

Ref: Despopoulos A, Silbernagl S. Color Atlas of Physiology. 120-150.

ANSWER 11

A. TRUE   B. FALSE   C. TRUE   D. TRUE   E. FALSE

PVR varies with lung volume in a U shaped curve, PVR is least at lung volumes ~ FRC. Histamine and 5HT increase PVR whereas prostacyclin reduces it (and is used in therapy for acute pulmonary hypertension). Anaemia reduces blood viscosity which decreases PVR and SVR.

Ref: Yentis, Hirsch, Smith. Anaesthesia A to Z. Butterworth-Heinemann

ANSWER 12

A. FALSE   B. TRUE   C. TRUE   D. FALSE   E. TRUE

Fetal bradycardia when a regional block is in place may be amenable to extension of the block if there is sufficient time and both maternal and obstetric consent. Maternal refusal, bleeding and a low platelet count are indications to avoid regional blocks. However many of the contraindications are relative and it is wise to liaise with the obstetricians in charge of the case and discuss and agree a management plan for the patient in question. Local sepsis, known allergy to local anaesthetics, coagulopathy, massive blood loss and maternal refusal are absolute contraindications to regional anaesthesia.

ANSWER 13

A. FALSE   B. TRUE   C. FALSE   D. TRUE   E. FALSE

Oliguria should be managed with a fluid challenge in the first instance. The use of a diuretic in hypovolaemia is associated with renal tubular damage. There is virtually no risk of infection with artificial colloids and so they should be used in preference to natural solutions if a volume effect is required; they are also less expensive than natural solutions, and the risk of an anaphylactic reaction is less. The infection risk from natural solutions includes hepatitis C, D and E and HIV. A volume of 1000 ml of HES will reduce the activity of factor VIII and prolongs PT. Anaphylaxis may require very large fluid replacement.

Ref: Nunn, Utting, Burnell Brown. General Anaesthesia. Butterworth-Heinemann

ANSWER 14

A. FALSE   B. TRUE   C. FALSE   D. TRUE   E. FALSE

Spontaneous electrical activity in the body are measured by the electrocardiogram (ECG), the electromyelogram (EMG) and the electroencephalogram (EEG). The signal voltage from the ECG and the EMG are greater than the EEG. The ECG is normally used with silver/silver chloride electrodes. Positive deflections in the ECG are due to current flow towards the positive electrode. Flow from the SA node to the atria occurs outwards in all directions so the P wave is positive in most electrode positions. In contrast the QRS complex moves in an ordered manner from the AV node toward the apex, and so the deflection depends on the electrode position. The amplifier of the ECG uses common mode rejection to increase the signal to noise ratio, whereas auditory evoked potentials are measured by summation of many individual signals in order to achieve the same aim.

Ref: Davis PD, Parbrook GD, Kenny GNC. Basic Physics and Measurement in Anaesthesia, 4th edn. Butterworth-Heinemann, 1995

ANSWER 15

A. FALSE   B. TRUE   C. FALSE   D. TRUE   E. FALSE

Iron, glucose and fat soluble vitamins are mostly absorbed in the jejunum.

Ref: Ganong WF. Review of Medical Physiology. Lange.

ANSWER 16

A. FALSE   B. TRUE   C. TRUE   D. TRUE   E. TRUE

Smooth muscle has slow pacemaker function. Bridges exist between cells. The action potential is generally spike-like with a duration of about 50 ms (skeletal = 10 ms, cardiac = 200 ms). It is followed by a slow rising contraction starting c. 150 ms later and peaking after 500 ms. Hence the state of constant partial contraction or tone found in smooth muscle.

Ref: Despopoulos A, Silbernagl S. Color Atlas of Physiology, 22-49

ANSWER 17

A. TRUE   B. TRUE   C. TRUE   D. FALSE   E. TRUE

Carbon dioxide lasers are used for superficial lesions, but need a helium laser as an aiming guide as the light produced is infra-red and not in the visible spectrum. Argon lasers are used in ophthalmology and neodymium-YAG lasers are used for their deeper penetration.

Ref: Blunt MC, Urquhart JC. The Anaesthesia Viva: Physics, Measurement, Safety and Clinical Anaesthesia. Greenwich Medical Media, 1996

ANSWER 18

A. FALSE   B. TRUE   C. FALSE   D. TRUE   E. FALSE

Dipalmitoylphosphatidylcholine is a phospholipid found in lung surfactant. It alters surface tension within the alveolus reducing atelectasis and pulmonary oedema. Surface tension varies according to alveolar size. Patchy atelectasis secondary to CP bypass is associated with decreased surfactant production.

Ref: Ganong WF. Review of Medical Physiology. Lange. Ch34.

ANSWER 19

A. FALSE B. TRUE C. FALSE D. FALSE E. FALSE

It does not have hydroxyl substitution of the benzene ring, and therefore cannot properly be called a catecholamine. It has some direct effect on receptors and exhibits effects in reserpine treated humans. It can exist in four isomeric forms but the only active one is the l-form. Ephedrine is supplied as the racaemic mixture or simply in the l-form.

ANSWER 20

A. TRUE B. TRUE C. TRUE D. FALSE E. FALSE

Allopurinol potentiates the action of warfarin by decreasing the rate of warfarin metabolism. Barbiturates decrease the action of warfarin by accelerating its metabolism via induction of hepatic microsomal enzymes.

ANSWER 21

A. TRUE B. TRUE C. FALSE D. FALSE E. TRUE

In order to minimise distortion the natural frequency of the monitoring system must be greater than that required for the harmonics of the input waveform (Fourier analysis breaks complex waves down into a fundamental frequency and its harmonics). In order to do this the equipment should use short, stiff-walled wide catheter tubing, with no connectors and no bubbles.

Damping (a reduction of the speed in which changes in the input pressure are shown in the output) leads to distortion of the waveform if it is either too large or too small. Bubbles and clots in the cannula will cause over-damping.

Ref: Urquhart JC, Blunt MC. The Anaesthesia Viva: Physiology, Pharmacology and Statistics, Greenwich Medical Media, 1996

ANSWER 22

A. TRUE B. FALSE C. FALSE D. FALSE E. FALSE

Cricoid pressure at 40 N is regarded as effective, but should be released if active vomiting takes place because of the risk of oesophageal rupture. The definitive means of ensuring correct placement is by capnography; misting may occur with oesophageal placement. Alfentanil does indeed reduce the pressor response, but no sedatives should be used in the rapid sequence induction as classically described. Neither should manual inflations be used, as this may inflate the stomach and increase the risk of vomiting; pre-oxygenation serves to ensure adequate oxygenation for the duration of the process of intubation.

ANSWER 23

A. TRUE B. FALSE C. FALSE D. FALSE E. FALSE

The CVP is a convenient measurement that may be used in assessing cardiac performance and circulating volume. It is not however a reliable indicator of left ventricular function, reflecting right heart function instead. Furthermore it is possible to develop pulmonary oedema with a normal CVP. The catheter should be placed in the superior vena cava as there is an increased incidence of thrombi forming on catheters in the right atrium. Measurements are either in mmHg if a transducer is used, or in cmH_2O if a saline manometer is used. 5 mmHg is equal to 6.5 cmH_2O.

Ref: Faust RJ (ed) Anesthesiology Review, 2nd edn. Churchill Livingstone, 1994

ANSWER   24

A. TRUE   B. TRUE   C. FALSE   D. TRUE   E. FALSE

Vagal stimulation increases insulin secretion, gastrin secretion, gastric acid secretion and bile production. It also causes bronchoconstriction thus reducing anatomical and therefore physiological dead space.

Ref: Ganong WF. Review of Medical Physiology. Lange.

ANSWER   25

A. FALSE   B. FALSE   C. FALSE   D. TRUE   E. TRUE

Hyoscine is a plant alkaloid resembling atropine. It has central and peripheral effects, which include sedative, anti-emetic and anti-sialogogue actions. Only 1% is excreted unchanged. It may paradoxically produce central stimulation, especially in the elderly.

ANSWER   26

A. FALSE   B. FALSE   C. FALSE   D. TRUE   E. TRUE

Causes of a fall in measured end-tidal carbon dioxide include:

Reduced production of carbon dioxide (shivering increases production of carbon dioxide)

Reduced transfer of the carbon dioxide from the tissues to the lungs (e.g. cardiac arrest)

Increased ventilation (endobroncheal intubation may cause no change or reduced ventilation)

Measurement of the respiratory dead space (e. g. extreme hypoventilation where the carbon dioxide containing alveolar gases do not reach the sampling tubing or chamber)

Inadequacies within the machine itself or its sample transfer system

An inadequate fresh gas flow (e.g. due to the N_2O failure) will cause rebreathing and a rise in end-tidal carbon dioxide.

Ref: Dorsch JA, Dorsch SE.   Understanding Anesthesia Equipment; Construction, Care and Complications, 2nd edn. Williams & Wilkins, 1984

ANSWER   27

A. FALSE   B. TRUE   C. FALSE   D. TRUE   E. TRUE

Understanding laminar flow is fundamental to the anaesthetist. Laminar flow may be considered to consist of numerous concentric tubes of fluid sliding relative to their neighbours. This allows the least resistance to flow, and the flow is least at the peripheries and greatest at the centre. Obviously the resistance to flow relates to the ease with which the concentric tubes can slide over each other - this is the viscosity. The density of the fluid is irrelevant in laminar flow (unlike turbulent flow). Laminar flow obeys the Hagen-Poiseuille law:

Flow = pi x radius(4) x pressure gradient / (8 x length x viscosity)

Ref: Mushin WM, Jones PL. Physics for the Anaesthetist, 4th edn. Blackwell Scientific Publications, 1987

ANSWER 28

A. FALSE   **B. TRUE**   **C. FALSE**   **D. FALSE**   **E. FALSE**

Peripheral chemoreceptors are located in the carotid and aortic bodies. The carotid body is the prime O_2 sensory organ. Ventilation is predominantly controlled by central chemoreceptors in the medulla which respond to a rise in $PaCO_2$ and CSF pH.

Ref: Despopoulos A, Silbernagl S. Color Atlas of Physiology. 78-108.

ANSWER 29

A. FALSE   **B. TRUE**   **C. TRUE**   **D. FALSE**   **E. FALSE**

Lipolysis is stimulated via beta receptors. Insulin release is actually inhibited by alpha receptor stimulation but stimulated via beta receptors. Bronchodilation is a beta 2 effect. Other alpha 1 effects include vasoconstriction.

Ref: Despopoulos A, Silbernagl S. Color Atlas of Physiology, 50-59

ANSWER 30

A. TRUE   **B. TRUE**   **C. FALSE**   **D. FALSE**   **E. FALSE**

A small proportion of the cardiac output reaches the lungs via the bronchial circulation. 1 kPa = c. 7.5 mmHg giving a mean pulmonary arterial pressure of 15 mmHg. Zone 1 is the apical third of the lung where PA >PA >Pv. Therefore blood flow occurs during systole. Pulmonary blood flow is maximal in zone 3 at the lung bases where PA >Pv >PA. V/Q ratios vary throughout the normal lung, being greater at the apex than the base. An average minute ventilation of 5.25 litres and a perfusion of roughly 5 l/min gives an overall V/Q ratio of c.1. Shunt leads to a V/Q ratio tending towards zero, dead space leads to a V/Q ratio that approaches infinity.

Ref: Despopoulos A, Silbernagl S. Color Atlas of Physiology, 94

ANSWER 31

A. FALSE   **B. TRUE**   **C. TRUE**   **D. TRUE**   **E. TRUE**

The Tec 4 is a plenum type vaporiser that is temperature and flow compensated (the former by using of bimetallic strip). It has a metal wick in the vaporisation chamber to help improve vaporisation. It has a Selectatec mount that helps stop the inadvertent use of two vaporisers at the same time. it also has a keyed filling mechanism to help prevent incorrect filling. According to COSHH (control of substances hazardous to health) guidelines filling of all vaporisers should be performed in a fume cupboard with a spill tray.

Ref: Davey A, Moyle JTB, Ward CS. Ward's Anaesthetic Equipment, 3rd edn. W.B. Saunders, 1992

ANSWER 32

A. FALSE   **B. FALSE**   **C. FALSE**   **D. FALSE**   **E. FALSE**

Remifentanil is a fentanyl derivative with an ester linkage. It is a pure mu receptor agonist, with a speed of onset similar to alfentanil. Clearance is not affected by pseudocholinesterase deficiency, its ultra-short action being the result of rapid breakdown of the ester linkage by non-specific tissue and plasma esterases. Although the main metabolic product of ester hydrolysis is excreted by the kidneys, it has a very low potency. Remifentanil is formulated in glycine, an inhibitory neuropeptide, and its use spinally or extradurally is not therefore recommended.

Ref: British Journal of Anaesthesia. 1996 76: 341-343.

ANSWER   33

A. FALSE   B. TRUE   C. TRUE   D. TRUE   E. FALSE

The muscle spindle is a fusiform capsule of connective tissue containing about 10 intrafusal striated muscle fibres. The middle of the spindle is surrounded by a spiral of nerve endings which register the degree of stretch of the muscle to the spinal cord via A-alpha fibres. The stretch reflex is thus initiated. Intrafusal fibre contraction may be initiated by gamma motorneurone stimulation leading to an altered response by the muscle spindle.

Ref: Ganong WF. Review of Medical Physiology. Lange, Ch6

ANSWER   34

A. FALSE   B. TRUE   C. FALSE   D. FALSE   D. TRUE

The A and B antigens are inherited as Mendelian dominants. The blood group of the man's children depends on their mother's blood group as well. His father may well have been O+ if his mother was group B or AB. If the mother is B+ his children could still be O+. The rarest blood group is AB-. Group O blood is the universal donor.

Ref: Ganong WF. Review of Medical Physiology. Lange. Ch27.

ANSWER   35

A. TRUE   B. TRUE   C. FALSE   D. FALSE   E. FALSE

Moclobemide is a reversible MAOI with no anti-emetic activity. Phenytoin has nausea and vomiting as a principle side effect.

Ref: BNF 1996

ANSWER   36

A. TRUE   B. TRUE   C. TRUE   D. TRUE   E. TRUE

The above all represent experimental or research techniques. The standard bed-side technique is thermodilution using a pulmonary artery catheter.

Ref: Yentis, Hirsch, Smith. Anaesthesia A to Z. Butterworth-Heinemann

ANSWER   37

A. FALSE   B. TRUE   C. FALSE   D. TRUE   E. FALSE

Thyroid hormones exert negative feedback on TSH production. They have a calorigenic action and increase oxygen dissociation by increasing RBC 2,3-DPG levels, and have a beta-like action on the heart.

Ref: Ganong WF. Review of Medical Physiology. Lange. Ch18.

ANSWER   38

A. TRUE   B. TRUE   C. FALSE   D. FALSE   E. TRUE

Aldosterone is a steroid hormone secreted from the zona glomerulosa and acts by altering mRNA synthesis at a nuclear level. It increases Na reabsorption from urine, sweat, saliva, and gastric juice. Release is in part stimulated by the renin-angiotensin system.

Ref: Ganong WF. Review of Medical Physiology. Lange, Ch20

ANSWER   39

A. TRUE   B. FALSE   C. TRUE   D. TRUE   E. TRUE

They are acetylcholinestase inhibitors, highly lipid soluble and so are readily absorbed across the skin. They phosphorylate the esteratic site of the acetylcholinesterase enzyme and are also inhibitors of plasma cholinesterase. The clinical features are those of a cholinergic crisis with both muscarinic and nicotinic effects. Spontaneous enzyme reactivation may occur but this is accelerated by pralidoxime if administered early. Other enzymes may also be phosphorylated. Respiratory failure may occur due to peripheral weakness, central depression and increased secretions.

Ref: Anaesthesia A to Z- An encyclopaedia of principles and practice.

ANSWER   40

A. FALSE   B. FALSE   C. FALSE   D. TRUE   E. TRUE

Mannitol is an alcohol and osmotic diuretic which is not absorbed from the GI tract. It does not enter cells. It is not metabolised in man. It should not be used in patients with cardiac failure due to the risk of circulatory overload. It is used in the treatment of cerebral oedema and in renoprotection in low output states or in association with acute liver failure.

PHYSICAL:

   10% = 550 mOsm/kg, 20% = 1100 mOsm/kg

DOSE:

   0.25-1 g/kg

Ref: Yentis, Hirsch, Smith. Anaesthesia A to Z . Butterworth-Heinemann

ANSWER   41

A. TRUE   B. FALSE   C. TRUE   D. TRUE   E. FALSE

Prostacyclin (PG12) is a potent inhibitor of platelet aggregation at a dose of approximately 5 ng/kg/min. The recommended dose range is 2-12 ng/kg/min. It is produced physiologically by vascular endothelium and has a half life of approximately 3 minutes. It is a vasodilator, which can result in hypotension. It is also used in ARDS and the treatment of pulmonary hypertension. It is useful as a platelet aggregation inhibitor for patients requiring haemodialysis who have heparin induced thrombocytopenia.

ANSWER   42

A. FALSE   B. FALSE   C. FALSE   D. TRUE   E. FALSE

Two compartment models are used to represent the fate of lipid soluble (high Vd) intravenous agents administered into the central vascular compartment. The second compartment represents redistributed agent residing in a deeper set of tissues which may redistribute back to the central compartment at a later time. Instead of plasma concentration declining exponentially in a simple first order fashion, it follows a more complex curve. The decline is very rapid at first as elimination from the plasma is augmented by simultaneous distribution from the central to deep compartments. The fall in concentration then becomes more gradual as less redistribution occurs. By the terminal portion of the curve fall in concentration is due almost entirely to elimination. This bi-exponential decay curve if plotted as log concentration against time can be broken down into two linear functions. A steep line of gradient alpha represents redistribution in the early phase, whereas the latter portion of shallower gradient beta represents elimination.

Ref: Nunn, Utting, Brown. General Anaesthesia. Butterworths.

ANSWER   43

A. TRUE   B. FALSE   C. FALSE   D. FALSE   E. FALSE

It is similar in structure to salbutamol and has a long, non-polar side chain which attaches itself to a site adjacent to the beta-receptor, allowing the active moeity to repeatedly stimulate the receptor thus accounting for its longer duration of action. It is fifteen times more potent than salbutamol at the beta-2 receptor, but four times less potent at the beta-1 receptor. It is long-acting requiring twice daily dosage. It has a relatively long onset time rendering it unsuitable for the acute treatment of asthma. Patients get tachyphylaxis to the unwanted side effects but not the bronchodilator properties.

Ref: Kaufmann, Taberner. Pharmacology in the Practice of Anaesthesia. Arnold, Chapter 19 part II

ANSWER   44

A. TRUE   B. TRUE   C. TRUE   D. TRUE   E. TRUE

Propofol is highly protein bound (97%). It has a volume of distribution at steady state of about 1000 litres. It is presented as an emulsion containing an isotonic 1% solution. Metabolism is in the liver with about 40% undergoing conjugation to a glucoronide and 60% metabolised to a quinol which is excreted as a glucoronide and sulphate. The metabolic clearance exceeds hepatic blood flow, suggesting extra-hepatic sites of metabolism. Only about 0.3% is excreted unchanged. A quinol metabolite is responsible for the discolouration of urine. It is safe in both MH and porphyria. About 15% of patients develop excitatory movements on induction. A fat overload syndrome, with hyperlipidaemia, and fatty infiltration of heart, liver, kidneys and lungs can follow prolonged infusion.

Ref: Nimmo, Rowbotham, Smith: Anaesthesia: chapter 6

ANSWER   45

A. FALSE   B. TRUE   C. TRUE   D. FALSE   E. TRUE

Once injected into the body where the pH rises above 4 the imidazole ring closes and the compound becomes lipid soluble; more so in fact that diazepam. Its elimination half life does not increase significantly in oliguric renal failure: it is largely hydroxylated by the liver.

Ref: Anesthesiology 1985; 62:310

ANSWER 46

A. TRUE   B. FALSE   C. FALSE   D. FALSE   E. FALSE

Sinus arrhythmia is the normal increase in heart rate on inspiration and decrease on expiration. It is marked in the young and athletes but still occurs in the elderly. It is vagally mediated and does not involve the stellate ganglion or the carotid sinus. It disappears on exertion.

Ref: Ganong WF. Review of Medical Physiology. Lange.

ANSWER 47

A. FALSE   B. TRUE   C. TRUE   D. TRUE   E. TRUE

The standard error of the mean equals the standard deviation divided by the number in the sample. The means of samples taken from a normally distributed population will themselves be normally distributed. The standard error of the mean of one sample is an estimate of the standard deviation that would be obtained from the means of a large number of samples drawn from that population.

Ref: Swinscow. Statistics at Square One. BMJ publications

ANSWER 48

A. TRUE   B. TRUE   C. TRUE   D. FALSE   E. TRUE

Bone consists of an organic matrix of calcium, phosphate, magnesium, sodium, and collagen. Undifferentiated cells at the bone surface can be activated by PTH and D hormone to form osteoclasts that bring about bone resorption. Alternatively their activity may be suppressed by calcitonin, leading to osteoblast transformation and new bone formation. Osteoblasts contain alkaline phosphatase that can create a high phosphate concentration locally, resulting in deposition of calcium when the solubility product is exceeded.

Ref: Despopoulos A, Silbernagl S. Color Atlas of Physiology, 232-271

ANSWER 49

A. FALSE   B. FALSE   C. TRUE   D. FALSE   E. FALSE

It is made up with water to form 2.5% solution containing 25 mg/ml. Stored with 6% sodium carbonate in an atmosphere of nitrogen, and causes a baroreceptor mediated reflex tachycardia.

PHYSICAL:

pH 10.8, pKa 7.661% non ionised at pH 7.465–86% protein binding

Ref: Sasada, Smith. Drugs in Anaesthesia and Intensive Care

ANSWER 50

A. FALSE   B. FALSE   C. FALSE   D. TRUE   E. TRUE

Milrinone is a bipyridine derivative. Enoximone and piroximone are imidazolone derivatives. It is used in infusion form but has a terminal half life of 2.5 hours. A loading dose is required. 80% is excreted unchanged via the kidneys, and dose reductions are required when the creatinine clearance falls to less than 30 ml/min.

Ref: British Journal of Anaesthesia 1992; 68: 293-302

ANSWER 51

A. FALSE   B. FALSE   C. TRUE   D. FALSE   E. TRUE

The MAC of enflurane is 1.68 (isoflurane 1.15). It has been reported to have been associated with renal damage although the levels of fluoride ions required to cause high output renal failure are twice those recorded after even very prolonged administration of enflurane. Nevertheless it seems sensible to avoid its use in such patients. Renal damage may be associated with the local renal metabolism of some of the volatile agents with different isoenzymes of the cytochrome P_{450} system. This may account for some of the toxicity of methoxyflurane

Ref: Aitkenhead, Smith. Textbook of Anaesthesia. Churchill Livingstone

ANSWER 52

A. FALSE   B. TRUE   C. TRUE   D. FALSE   E. TRUE

Salbutamol and ritodrine are used in obstetric practice to inhibit premature labour (tocolysis by beta-2 receptor stimulation). Other agents which relax uterine tone include:

Volatile agents

Adrenaline (NB alpha effects may override this)

Intravenous anaesthetic agents, neuromuscular blockers and anticholinesterase inhibitors have no effect. Alcohol may have a direct relaxant action.

ANSWER 53

A. TRUE   B. FALSE   C. FALSE   D. TRUE   E. TRUE

Chassaignac's tubercle is the transverse process of C6, at the level of the Cricoid cartilage. The Stellate ganglion overlies this and is separated from it by the prevertebral fascia. The technique is used for relief of chronic pain which is sympathetically mediated but is not useful for surgical anaesthesia. A Horner's syndrome is inevitable if the block is carried out effectively as a sympathetic block ensues: miosis, enophthalmos, ptosis, flushed skin and congested nose. Among the complications are a subarachnoid block, phrenic nerve and recurrent laryngeal nerve palsy; pneumothorax, though possible, is not as likely a complication as in brachial plexus blocks.

Ref: Nunn, Utting, Burnell Brown. General Anaesthesia. Butterworth-Heinemann

ANSWER 54

A. TRUE   B. FALSE   C. TRUE   D. TRUE   E. TRUE

The carotid bodies are peripheral chemoreceptors situated above the carotid bifurcation. They receive proportionally the highest blood flow in the body (2000 ml / 100 g / min) and their O_2 demands are entirely met by dissolved O_2. They respond to changes in O_2 tension (either due to reduced PaO_2 or reduced cardiac output) rather than oxygen content, hence do not alter discharge rate in anaemia and carbon monoxide poisoning.

Ref: Ganong WF. Review of Medical Physiology. Lange. Ch36.

ANSWER 55

A. FALSE   B. FALSE   C. FALSE   D. TRUE   E. TRUE

With the first gasp and lung volume expansion the PVR falls to < 20% of the pre-birth value, LA pressure rises and the foramen ovale closes (but does not fuse for ~ 48 hours).

Ref: Ganong WF. Review of Medical Physiology. Lange. Ch32.

ANSWER 56

A. TRUE   B. FALSE   C. TRUE   D. FALSE   E. FALSE

Approximately 5% of sevoflurane is metabolised. Despite close structural similarities with desflurane, the two have markedly different physical properties. The low blood:gas (0.67) solubility and minimal airway irritation allow for smooth and rapid induction. It is degraded by soda-lime and baralyme to produce so-called compound A (and to a lesser extent compound B). This is a heat dependant reaction and the FDA therefore recommend that it is not used in low flow anaesthesia with a fresh gas flow of less than 3 litres per minute.

Ref: Smith, Nathanson, White. Sevoflurane - A long awaited volatile anaesthetic. British Journal of Anasethesia 1996; 76: 435-445.

ANSWER 57

A. TRUE   B. TRUE   C. FALSE   D. FALSE   E. FALSE

It causes hypotension, but curiously causes umbilical artery spasm. Its action on uterine muscle is oestrogen dependent.

ANSWER 58

A. FALSE   B. FALSE   C. FALSE   D. FALSE   E. TRUE

Ingested iron is mostly in the ferric state, and only about 5% of ingested iron is absorbed. It is best absorbed in the ferrous state. A trace of iron is absorbed in the stomach but it is mostly absorbed in the jejunum.

Ref: Ganong WF. Review of Medical Physiology, Lange

ANSWER 59

A. TRUE   B. FALSE   C. TRUE   D. TRUE   E. TRUE

Carbamezepine causes facial abnormalities, IUGR, microcephaly & mental retardation. Increased incidence with increased dose. Incidence overall c. 1/300-2000 live births. Nitrous oxide has not been shown to cause fetal abnormalities. Phenytoin causes craniofacial abnormalities, growth retardation, limb and cardiac defects and mental retardation. Sodium valproate causes neural tube defects. In general the incidence of fetal abnormalities associated with anticonvulsants increases with increasing dose and with the use of more than one agent. Warfarin is teratogenic and women taking warfarin should be advised to stop it before the sixth week of pregnancy. In the last trimester warfarin crosses the placenta and may cause fetal /maternal haemorrhage. Heparin should therefore be used instead particularly in the first and third trimesters. Difficult decisions may have to be taken in women with prosthetic heart valves.

ANSWER 60

A. TRUE   B. FALSE   C. TRUE   D. TRUE   E. FALSE

A mole is a basic SI unit defined as the amount of particles equal to that of 0.012 kg of carbon 12. It contains Avagadros number of particles 6.023 x 10$^{(23)}$. A mole of gas occupies a constant volume (22.4 litres at s.t.p.)

Ref: Strickland DAP. S I Units. In: Scurr C, Feldman S, Soni N (Eds) Scientific Foundations of Anaesthesia; The Basis of Intensive Care, 4th edn. Heinemann Medical Books, 1990, pp 1-9

ANSWER 61

A. FALSE   B. TRUE   C. FALSE   D. FALSE   E. FALSE

The dibucaine number refers to the degree of inhibition of plasma cholinesterase by dibucaine in vitro; the degree of inhibition is reduced in the presence of an abnormal enzyme. Malignant hyperpyrexia is an autosomal dominant condition investigated by muscle biopsy; suxamethonium apnoea is transmitted as an autosomal recessive condition. Blood products should not be used to provide missing enzyme because of the risk of disease transmission, and because the situation will resolve with time. The patient should be sedated and ventilated until neuromuscular function returns.

ANSWER 62

A. TRUE   B. FALSE   C. FALSE   D. TRUE   E. TRUE

There is a large list of drugs that may precipitate an attack of hepatic porphyria. The candidate is advised to look up the more common anaesthetic drugs in the reference.

Ref: Nimmo, Rowbotham, Smith. Anaesthesia, Blackwell, chapter 54

ANSWER 63

A. TRUE   B. FALSE   C. TRUE   D. FALSE   E. FALSE

Antiemetics include:

5HT antagonists (ondansetron) acting at 5HT3 receptors

Phenothiazines (prochlorperazine) acting at D2 receptors

Butyrophenones (droperidol) acting at D2 receptors

Antihistamines (cyclizine) acting at H1 receptors

Anticholinergics (hyoscine) acting at Ach receptors

Benzamides (metoclopramide) acting at D2 receptors

Metoclopramide acts centrally by blocking dopamine receptors at the chemoreceptor trigger zone, and peripherally by increasing lower oesophageal sphincter tone and enhancing gastric motility. Phenothiazines such as prochlorperazine are dopamine antagonists. Cyclizine is associated with a very low incidence of extrapyramidal side effects. The half-life of ondansetron is 3 hours.

ANSWER 64

A. FALSE   B. FALSE   C. TRUE   D. TRUE   E. FALSE

The highest risk is associated with cardiac failure and recent myocardial infarction. The index identifies high-risk patients, but does not predict outcome although 56% of those with a score over 25 died. It is specific (it only identifies at-risk patients) but poorly sensitive (it does not identify them all). Angina and hypertension were not included as risk factors although most people would regard them as such.

Ref: Goldman L et al, New England Journal of Medicine 297: 845-850

ANSWER 65

A. TRUE   B. TRUE   C. FALSE   D. TRUE   E. FALSE

The valsalva manoeuvre is forced expiration against a closed glottis following maximal inspiration. Middle ear pressure increases and the manoeuvre was originally described as a technique for expelling pus from the middle ear. At glottic closure there is a rise in intra-thoracic pressure causing a slight transient increase in blood pressure, however as venous return is reduced BP falls. This activates the baroreceptor reflex causing vasoconstriction and tachycardia, so BP rises to near normal. On opening the glottis intra-thoracic pressure suddenly falls thus BP falls, however this is rapidly corrected as venous return is restored. The heart rate drops and overshoots causing a bradycardia before returning to normal. The valsalva is useful as a bed-side test of autonomic function. With autonomic neuropathy you generally see a prolonged reduction in blood pressure throughout glottic closure, with an absence of changes in heart rate. The manoeuvre can also be used to terminate SVTs because of increased vagal tone upon glottic opening.

Ref: Yentis, Hirsch, Smith. Anaesthesia A to Z. Butterworth-Heinemann

ANSWER 66

A. FALSE   B. FALSE   C. TRUE   D. FALSE   E. FALSE

Hypokalaemia is a consequence of beta-agonists and steroids. Pulsus paradoxus refers to blood pressure and not pulse rate changes with breathing in severe asthmatics. Ephedrine is not used in the treatment of asthma in the UK but all the other drugs are used. Chest X-ray is unlikely to be informative and blood gases should be performed only on severely ill patients, who would not be suitable for elective surgery in any case.

ANSWER 67

A. TRUE   B. TRUE   C. FALSE   D. FALSE   E. TRUE

Verapamil inhibits the slow Ca-channel in the A-V node, increases the effective refractory period but does not cause long Q-T. Sotalol, a beta blocker, posesses class III activity, and both quinidine and disopyramide have class 1A actions with mild class III activity prolonging the cardiac action potential and hence the Q-T interval. Flecainide, a class IC antiarhythmic agent does not directly prolong the Q-T interval.

Ref: Opie L. Drugs for the Heart. Saunders

ANSWER 68

A. FALSE   B. TRUE   C. FALSE   D. TRUE   E. FALSE

The LMWHs do not bind ATIII and thrombin simultaneously; They cannot catalyse the inhibition of thrombin but do effect the inhibition of activated IX ,X, XI and XII by ATIII. They thus have less effect on platelet activity than heparin. They have a longer duration of action than heparin. Protamine is usually given in a dose of 1 mg for every 100 u (1 mg) when a loading dose has been given for example in cardiac surgery.

Ref: British Journal of Anaesthesia 1995; 75(5): 622

ANSWER 69

A. FALSE   B. TRUE   C. FALSE   D. TRUE   E. TRUE

The infra-red absorption spectrometer is the most common capnometer seen in theatre at present. It has a short response time (50–100 ms or faster) which allows it to be used on a breath-to-breath basis. The CO_2 analyser relies on Beer's law that states that the absorption of a substance is exponentially proportional to its concentration. The CO_2 analyser measures absorption in the infra-red range at 4.3 µm. A broad spectrum emitter is used and the light passes through a filter before being slit into two paths. One goes to a control chamber and the other to the sample chamber. These have sapphire windows as glass is relatively opaque to infra-red light. A 'chopper wheel' allows light to pass to only one chamber at a time. The light then passes to the detector and the CO_2 is calculated from the difference in the absorption between the sample and the control.

Ref: Tremper KK, Wahr JA. Advances in respiratory monitoring. In: Sanford TJ (Ed) Clinical Issues in Monitoring. W.B. Saunders, 1994, pp 261-276

ANSWER 70

A. TRUE   B. TRUE   C. FALSE   D. FALSE   E. FALSE

The Nernst equation allows calculation of the equilibrium potential between the inner and outer surfaces of a cell membrane. $E = (RT/(Fz))(\ln([x]out/[x]in))$. Positivity or negativity of the potential is therefore also partially dependent on z, the ionic charge, as well as the intracellular:extracellular concentration ratio. In the resting cell $E_k = -90$ mV.

Ref: Despopoulos A, Silbernagl S. Color Atlas of Physiology. 1-17.

ANSWER 71

A. FALSE   B. TRUE   C. TRUE   D. FALSE   E. TRUE

Scavenging is a requirement under the 'control of substances hazardous to health' (COSHH). It may be active or passive, the latter including the Cardiff Aldasorber containing activated charcoal. This is effective for volatile anaesthetic agents but of no value for scavenging nitrous oxide. Scavenging systems are attached by 30 mm fittings, that are not interchangeable with the breathing system fittings. These should be fitted with valves to ensure the negative pressure developed is kept below 0.5 cmH_2O and the positive pressure below 10 cmH_2O. The discharge should be outside away from areas where personnel commonly work.

Ref: Davey A, Moyle JTB, Ward CS. Ward's Anaesthetic Equipment, 3rd edn. W.B. Saunders., 1992

ANSWER 72

A. FALSE   B. TRUE   C. FALSE   D. FALSE   E. TRUE

Human lung compliance is approximately 200 mls/ cmH_2O, whereas total thoracic compliance is about 85 ml/ cmH_2O. Static compliance can be measured using a spirometer and a simple water manometer though it is more usual to use an electrical transducer these days. In IPPV tidal volume depends on total thoracic compliance and in practice may also be influenced by severe airway resistance. Dynamic compliance is measured at different points in the respiratory cycle (usually end-inspiratory and end-expiratory) when no gas is flowing. Compliance is related to body size hence specific compliance is often quoted (compliance/FRC).

Ref: Nunn JF. Applied Respiratory Physiology. Butterworth.-Heinemann

ANSWER 73

A. FALSE   B. TRUE   C. FALSE   D. FALSE   E. TRUE

The average MW is 35 000. The reactions are anaphylactoid and occur in <0.15% of patients: prior exposure is not necessary. There is no evidence for an increased incidence of pulmonary oedema compared with any synthetic or non-synthetic colloid. Gelofusin is succinylated whereas haemaccel is urea linked. They have a short vascular retention time of about 4 hours.

Ref: Anaesthesia 1987; 47: 998

ANSWER 74

A. FALSE   B. TRUE   C. TRUE   D. FALSE   E. FALSE

The synaptic cleft is 30-50 nm wide. Summation of excitatory postsynaptic potentials may be both spatial and temporal. Normal synaptic delay is 0.5 ms. IPSPs are hyperpolarising and EPSPs depolarising by definition.

Ref: Ganong WF. Review of Medical Physiology. Lange.

ANSWER 75

A. FALSE   B. FALSE   C. TRUE   D. TRUE   E. FALSE

The 'physiological anaemia of pregnancy' is due to plasma expansion exceeding red cell expansion. The blood becomes hypercoagulable with increases in fibrinogen and factors VII, IX, X and XII. Platelet count and FDPs increase.

Ref: Yentis, Hirsch, Smith. Anaesthesia A to Z. Butterworth-Heinemann.

ANSWER 76

A. TRUE   B. FALSE   C. TRUE   D. TRUE   E. FALSE

A population is a group of subjects sharing a parameter, all males in a town, or all subjects in a control group. The Chi-squared test can only be used for nominal data; yes/no, dead/alive. A value of $p<0.05$ is accepted in medicine as being significant, showing as it does, that there is only a 1:20 chance of the null hypothesis obtaining. A value of $p<0.001$ is very highly significant.

ANSWER 77

A. TRUE   B. FALSE   C. FALSE   D. TRUE   E. TRUE

The amount of oxygen, nitrous oxide and anaesthetic agent required by the body for oxygenation and anaesthesia is related to the partial pressure of these in the trachea. For convenience the more easily measured concentration or fraction is used, and the barometric pressure is assumed to be constant. At high altitude the barometric pressure is reduced. The partial pressure of anaesthetic agent that is delivered by the vaporiser is constant at differing barometric pressures, so the concentration dialled into the apparatus will have the same clinical effect as the SVP is unchanged if the temperature is the same. However the fraction (%) actually delivered will be higher than the dialled value as the absolute pressure in the enviroment is lower. Furthermore to get the same partial pressure of oxygen at lower barometric pressure requires a higher inspired fraction, and the same inspired fraction of nitrous oxide will provide a lower partial pressure and so a reduced effect. This can be confusing and it is advisable to read the reference.

Ref: Dorsch JA, Dorsch SE. Understanding Anesthesia Equipment; Construction, Care and Complications, 2nd edn. Wlliams & Wilkins, 1984

ANSWER 78

A. TRUE   B. TRUE   C. TRUE   D. FALSE   E. TRUE

The apparent volume of distribution (Vd) is defined as the volume of fluid required to contain the total amount (Q) of drug in the body at the same concentration as that present in the plasma (Cp). Volume of distribution Vd = Q/Cp.

Drugs confined to the plasma compartment will have a small volume of distribution while those with high lipid solubility (and a low plasma concentration due to redistribution) appear to have a large volume of distribution. It depends on the partition coefficient (determined by the degree of ionisation), regional blood flow and the degree of protein/ tissue binding.

ANSWER 79

A. TRUE   B. FALSE   C. FALSE   D. FALSE   E. TRUE

The pulse oximeter measures light absorption 30 times a second in order to be able to calculate the pulsatile component of the absorption. Original oximeters used a filtered light source but this was bulky and has been superseded by the use of two light-emitting diodes (LEDs). Errors may occur if there are pulsatile elements that are not due to arterial blood (e.g. venous pulsation in tricuspid incompetence) or abnormal elements within the arterial blood itself (carboxyhaemoglobin has an absorption spectrum similar to oxyhaemoglobin and leads to a falsely high SpO_2 - by as much as 10-15% in heavy smokers).

Ref: Sykes MK, Vickers MD, Hull CJ. Principles of Measurement and Monitoring in Anaesthesia and Intensive Care, 3rd edn. Blackwell Scientific Publishers, 1991

ANSWER 80

A. TRUE   B. TRUE   C. FALSE   D. FALSE   E. FALSE

The basic Systéme International d' Units is the international basis for the definition of measurement. It consists of seven units: Metre, Kilogram, Second, Ampere, Kelvin, Mole, Candela.

Ref: Strickland DAP. S I Units. In: Scurr C, Feldman S, Soni N. (Eds) Scientific Foundations of Anaesthesia; The Basis of Intensive Care, 4th edn. Heinemann Medical Books, 1990, pp 1-9

ANSWER 81

A. TRUE   B. TRUE   C. FALSE   D. FALSE   E. TRUE

JVP c wave is caused by isovolumetric intraventricular pressure rise transmitted across a closed tricuspid valve to the SVC. The 1st heart sound is caused by closure of the mitral and tricuspid valves and must therefore precede isovolumetric contraction. Normal SV=70-90 ml and ESV=50 ml. Duration of systole decreases from 0.3 s at HR 65 to 0.16 s at HR 200 but changes in diastolic time are more marked.

Ref: Ganong WF. Review of Medical Physiology. Lange, Ch29

ANSWER 82

A. FALSE   B. TRUE   C. FALSE   D. TRUE   E. FALSE

A circle is designed for low-flow anaesthesia (which is defined as less than 3 l/min) and although it is intended for use at flows below this, higher flows are required when initiating anaesthesia and when purging the system. The minute ventilation when using a minute volume divider is set by the flowmeters on the anaesthetic machine.

ANSWER 83

A. TRUE   B. TRUE   C. FALSE   D. FALSE   E. FALSE

A nerve stimulator designed to assess neuromuscular blockade should be able to deliver a stimulus of 60-70 mA. Tetany can be sustained by normal patients for at least 5 seconds in the absence of neuromuscular block. Post-tetanic facilitation and fade are features of non-depolarising block. Prolonged suxamethonium blockade (either due to repeated doses or suxamethonium apnoea) may develop features of non-depolarising block, including fade and post-tetanic facilitation. This is called dual or phase II block. Head lift is an extremely good clinical indicator of recovery of neuromuscular function.

Ref: Faust RJ (ed). Anesthesiology Review, 2nd edn. Churchill Livingstone, 1994

ANSWER 84

A. TRUE   B. FALSE   C. FALSE   D. TRUE   E. TRUE

Essentially any drug that is metabolised by microsomal liver enzymes should be avoided since the activity of d-aminolaevulinic acid synthetase is increased.

Ref: Watkins J, Levy CJ. Guide to Immediate Anaesthetic Reactions. Butterworth-Heinemann

ANSWER 85

A. TRUE   B. TRUE   C. FALSE   D. TRUE   E. TRUE

Viral infection usually causes a lymphocytosis and not a neutropaenia.

Ref: Hoffbran, Pettit. Essential Haematology. Blackwell.

ANSWER 86

A. TRUE   B. TRUE   C. FALSE   D. FALSE   E. TRUE

Deoxygenated blood arrives at the placenta from the fetus via the two umbilical arteries and returns oxygenated via the single umbilical vein. Uterine (and hence maternal placental) blood flow is directly related to mean uterine perfusion pressure and inversely related to uterine vascular resistance (which is increased by hyperventilation, stress and vasopressors.)

Ref: Yentis, Hirsch, Smith. Anaesthesia A to Z. Butterworth-Heinemann.

ANSWER 87

A. FALSE   B. TRUE   C. TRUE   D. FALSE   E. FALSE

Hydralazine is predominantly an arteriolar dilator which leads to a reduced systemic vascular resistance and associated tachycardia. It is associated with an increase in cardiac output and cerebral blood flow. It may result in a lupus-like syndrome after chronic usage. Peripheral neuropathies and blood dyscrasias have also been reported.

ANSWER 88

A. FALSE   B. TRUE   C. TRUE   D. FALSE   E. TRUE

Erythromycin is a macrolide antibiotic effective against gram positive AEROBES. It is both bacteriostatic and bactericidal and inhibits peptide translocase by binding to the bacterial ribosome. It may potentiate the effects of warfarin, theophylline and digoxin. It increases gut motility and thus reduces gut transit time. It has been used to attempt to stimulate absorption from the gut in ITU in patients with an ileus.

Ref: Sasada, Smith. Drugs in Anaesthesia and Intensive Care.

ANSWER 89

A. TRUE   B. FALSE   C. FALSE   D. TRUE   E. TRUE

If a drug is 50% protein bound, and this is decreased to 48%, the free drug concentration will increase by 4%. On the other hand, if the drug is 98% bound and this decreases to 96%, the free drug concentration doubles from 2% to 4% of total. This is a 100% not 2% increase in free drug concentration. Drugs which are extensively bound and which are poorly extracted by the liver will display an increased clinical effect if displaced as free drug. Both Diazepam and midazolam are extensively protein bound. Drug pKa is in this case irrelevent.

Ref: Nunn, Utting, Brown. General Anaesthesia. Butterworths.

ANSWER 90

A. TRUE   B. TRUE   C. FALSE   D. TRUE   E. FALSE

A body plethysmograph and an oesophageal balloon may be used to measure intrapleural pressure. Measurements of pressure and volume may then be plotted against one another to give pressure:volume compliance loops. Dynamic compliance can be calculated from the slope of the line joining no-flow points at maximum inspiration and expiration. The width of the loop indicates airway resistance. The area within it corresponds to the work of breathing ($P \times V = N/m^2 \times m^3 = Nm = $ Joules). The pressure gradient generated and the time component involved, make the plethysmograph unsuitable for measuring FEV_1. Gas exchange can be assessed by ABG analysis and non-invasively by measurement of the transfer factor for carbon monoxide by the single breath or steady state method.

Ref: Aitkenhead, Smith. Textbook of Anaesthesia. Churchill Livingstone, Ch2

Exam 5

QUESTION 1

At most sympathetic postganglionic nerve endings

A. Dopamine is formed by N-methylation of tyramine
B. 70% of released noradrenaline is actively reabsorbed into presynaptic nerve endings
C. Extraneuronal breakdown of noradrenaline occurs principally via monoamine oxidase
D. Down regulation of noradrenergic activity is mediated by post-synaptic alpha 2 receptors
E. The second messenger at alpha 1 receptors is cGMP

QUESTION 2

Iron

A. Is present in the plasma as ferritin
B. 95% of whole body iron is in haemoglobin
C. Is present in the plasma as transferrin
D. In iron deficiency, total transferrin is increased
E. In iron deficiency, transferrin saturation is reduced

QUESTION 3

A grade 1 protein poor diet (Kwashiorkor) is associated with

A. A fall in urea excretion
B. A fall in creatinine excretion
C. A urea nitrogen excretion of approximately 14 g/day
D. Increased uric acid excretion
E. Anaemia

QUESTION 4

Temperature measurement

A. A mercury thermometer is suitable for measuring temperatures from −30°C to at least 200°C
B. A resistance thermometer is normally used in a Wheatstone bridge configuration
C. A thermistor has a metal oxide electrode whose resistance changes exponentially with increasing temperature
D. The calibration of a thermistor is resistant to heat sterilisation
E. A thermocouple relies on the Seebeck effect to measure temperature change

QUESTION 5

Prazocin

  A. Is useful in the first-line treatment of malignant hypertension
  B. Achieves its action by binding to alpha-2 adrenoceptors
  C. Does not provoke a reflex tachycardia
  D. Should be used with caution in patients receiving concomitant diuretic therapy
  E. Is associated with first dose hypotension

QUESTION 6

Carotid sinus massage

  A. Causes reflex inhibition of the vasomotor centre
  B. Activates the cardio-inhibitory centre
  C. Can be complicated by ventricular tachycardia
  D. Reduces cerebral blood flow
  E. Is still effective in an anaesthetised patient

QUESTION 7

Carbimazole

  A. Is metabolised to methimazole, the active drug
  B. Acts by preventing release of triiodothyronine
  C. Crosses the placenta to cause fetal hypothyroidism
  D. Is contra-indicated in breast-feeding
  E. Clinical effects of inhibition of thyroid function are seen within 24 hours

QUESTION 8

During diving

  A. Ambient pressure increases by 1 atmosphere for every 20 m depth in sea water
  B. Ambient pressure increase in fresh water will be less than at an equivalent depth of sea water
  C. Normal air at 15m depth is an hypoxic mixture
  D. Fatal air embolism may occur if a snorkel diver does not exhale whilst surfacing rapidly
  E. High pressure nervous syndrome is associated with deep dives

QUESTION 9

Concerning elimination of drugs

  A. Alcohol metabolism is a first order process
  B. At low concentrations thiopentone elimination is a first order process
  C. At high concentrations phenytoin elimination is a zero order process
  D. Desflurane is eliminated as a second order process
  E. Fentanyl metabolism is a zero order process

QUESTION 10

The following are true

A. Fourier analysis is the break-down of a complex waveform into a sine wave and its harmonics
B. Because of Boyle's Law a graph of pressure against volume would be a parabola
C. The graph of the gas pressure from an oxygen cylinder discharging at constant temperature would be of the form $P = P_0 \cdot e^{(-kt)}$
D. An exponential function can be made linear by log transformation
E. The time constant of an exponential function is the time taken for the function to fall by 36.8% of its original value

QUESTION 11

Concerning 2,3-DPG

A. It is formed from a product of glycolysis
B. Binds the alpha chains of deoxyhaemoglobin
C. Is poorly bound by foetal haemoglobin
D. Its red cell concentration is increased by increased circulating thyroid hormones
E. An increased concentration increases oxygen utilisation by cells

QUESTION 12

The following are recognised complications of phenytoin

A. Tremor
B. Blood dyscrasias
C. Corneal deposits
D. Acne
E. Gastric irritation

QUESTION 13

The following antibiotics exert their action by destruction of the bacterial cell wall

A. Teicoplanin
B. Cephalosporins
C. The macrolides
D. Metronidazole
E. Flucloxacillin

QUESTION 14

The following cause rebreathing of carbon dioxide

A. Channels within the soda lime
B. Disconnection at the endotracheal tube
C. Inadvertent bypassing of the soda lime absorber
D. Failure of the oxygen supply
E. Failure of the unidirectional valves in the circle system

QUESTION   15

In the normal human kidney

A. One would expect to find more than one million nephrons
B. Distal tubular cells do not possess brush borders
C. Proximal tubular cells possess fewer mitochondria than distal tubular cells
D. Only 20% of nephrons have a loop of Henle
E. The slit membrane of the Bowman's capsule has pores of 5 nm diameter

QUESTION   16

Concerning the side effects of tricyclic antidepressants

A. Desipramine produces fewer anticholinergic side effects than amitryptiline
B. ECG abnormalities include prolongation of the P-R interval and widening of the QRS complex
C. Orthostatic hypotension is relatively common
D. At therapeutic levels, sedation is rarely a problem
E. The pressor response to ephedrine is increased

QUESTION   17

The following are parametric tests

A. Cochrane's test
B. Fisher's exact test
C. Student's t-test
D. Spearman's rank correlation
E. Weber's test

QUESTION   18

According to the Hagen-Poiseuille equation

A. Flow varies inversely with the fourth power of the radius
B. Flow varies inversely with fluid density
C. Flow varies directly with pressure difference between the ends of the vessel
D. Haematocrit is likely to inversely affect blood flow
E. If the radius of a vessel is doubled, resistance will fall to less than 50% of its previous value.

QUESTION   19

The following drugs act as potassium sparing diuretics

A. Enalapril
B. Frusemide
C. Triamterene
D. Amiloride
E. Hydrochlorothiazide

QUESTION 20

The following are necessary for a fire to occur

A. Activation or initiation energy
B. Fuel
C. Air
D. An oxidising agent
E. Heat

QUESTION 21

The following are natural precursors of adrenaline

A. Noradrenaline
B. Glycine
C. Tyrosine
D. Dihydroxyphenylalanine
E. Dobutamine

QUESTION 22

Concerning preoperative assessment

A. Chest X-ray is a useful investigation in a patient who may have congestive cardiac failure (CCF)
B. Haemoglobin concentration (Hb) should be measured in all menstruating women presenting for elective anaesthesia
C. A low serum potassium may be present in a patient taking a loop diuretic
D. A single electrocardiogram (ECG) is helpful in identifying the presence of ischaemic heart disease
E. An echocardiogram is a useful investigation where an ejection systolic murmur is present

QUESTION 23

Tramadol

A. Is a controlled drug
B. Has an analgesic potency equal to that of morphine, without the respiratory depressant side effects
C. Produces its action solely via mu opioid receptors
D. Has an active metabolite O-desmethyl tramadol
E. Can be safely given to patients receiving monoamine oxidase inhibitors

QUESTION 24

Awareness under anaesthesia

A. The risk of awareness can be reduced with the use of a volatile agent monitor alarm adjusted to a value of 1 MAC

B. Has been described in conjunction with total intravenous anaesthesia (TIVA)

C. The PRST score assesses pressure, lacrimation, movement and sweating on a scale from 0 to 8

D. If awareness is suspected during the course of an anaesthetic, 10 mg midazolam will abolish the recollection of events

E. Awareness can reliably be detected by continuous measurement of the bispectral index (BSI)

QUESTION 25

The Siggaard-Anderson curve nomogram

A. Has PCO_2 on the vertical scale

B. Has pH on the horizontal scale

C. Determines standard bicarbonate content after plotting measured PCO_2 and pH of a blood gas sample

D. Plots base excess on a secondary x-axis

E. Allows estimation of the buffer base content

QUESTION 26

Definitions

A. A fluid is a substance that expands to occupy the space in which it is confined

B. Heat represents the average kinetic energy of a substance

C. Absolute zero is the point at which all molecular motion ceases

D. A vapour is a gas below its boiling point

E. 1 calorie is the energy provided by 1 mg of sugar

QUESTION 27

Prolonged vomiting may cause

A. Alkaline urine

B. Hypernatraemia

C. Hyperchloraemia

D. Hypokalaemia and acidic urine

E. Renal bicarbonate loss

QUESTION 28

Hypermagnesaemia may cause

A. Hypertension
B. Hyperreflexia
C. Hypercapnia
D. Tetany
E. Vomiting

QUESTION 29

Concerning immunoglobulins

A. IgM exists as a pentamer
B. IgA is secretory
C. IgM appears in breast milk
D. IgM crosses the placenta
E. IgE releases histamine and heparin from mast cells

QUESTION 30

Gamma-aminobutyric acid (GABA)

A. Is formed by the carboxylation of glutamate
B. Increases chloride ion conductance
C. Is an inhibitory neurotransmitter
D. Is found in the retina
E. Occurs as a pre-synaptic transmitter

QUESTION 31

Theophylline

A. Mainly produces bronchodilation by its action on adenosine receptors
B. Increases the force of diaphragmatic contraction in patients with COPD
C. Is a mild CNS depressant
D. Causes vasodilatation
E. Increases the release of catecholamines from the adrenal medulla.

QUESTION 32

Nitrous oxide

A. Is principally produced as a by product in the nylon industry
B. Inhibits methionine reductase
C. Causes an increase in sympathetic outflow
D. Is associated with post operative nausea and vomiting
E. Has no effect on pulmonary vascular resistance

QUESTION   33

Dextrans

A. Are polysaccharides made by the action of Leuconostoc mesenteroides on sucrose
B. Interfere with haemostasis
C. Can lead to acute renal failure due to blockage of renal tubules
D. Are associated with fewer allergic reactions than the gelatin plasma expanders
E. Have an average molecular weight of 11 0000

QUESTION   34

Remifentanil

A. Is a phenylpiperidine derivative.
B. Is a basic drug with a pKa value less than physiological pH
C. Is largely ionised at body pH rendering it water soluble
D. Is predominantly broken down by plasma esterases
E. Has a context-sensitive half-time that is independant of the duration of infusion.

QUESTION   35

The Manley ventilator

A. Is a flow generator
B. Is a minute volume divider
C. Is commonly used with a closed system
D. Does not need a ventilator disconnection device as any change of ventilation pattern can be heard
E. Contains 3 valves and 2 bellows

QUESTION   36

A capacitor

A. Is central to the function of a defibrillator
B. Is a way of storing current
C. Has a resistance to AC current flow that is independent of the frequency of the current
D. Has a capacitance measured in Farads (F)
E. May be thought of as two conductors separated by an insulator

QUESTION   37

Mannitol

A. Increases plasma osmolarity
B. Is contra-indicated in cardiac failure
C. Can be used in the management of fulminant hepatic failure
D. When used in the treatment of raised intra-cranial pressure, relies on its ability to cross the blood-brain barrier
E. Is administered in a dose of approximately 0.25-1 mg/kg

QUESTION 38

Captopril

   A. Produces an increase in plasma aldosterone and renin levels
   B. Is highly protein bound in the circulation
   C. Is excreted unchanged in the urine in significant amounts
   D. Is effective as a once daily dose
   E. May cause blood dyscrasias

QUESTION 39

Blood flow in the right coronary artery

   A. Is reduced by vagal stimulation
   B. Is increased by intra-coronary cyanide
   C. Is reduced to zero during ventricular systole
   D. Is increased by intra-coronary potassium
   E. Can be measured by applying the Kety method

QUESTION 40

The inverse stretch reflex

   A. Induces relaxation of antagonistic muscle groups
   B. Is mediated by the Golgi tendon organ
   C. May be induced by passive stretch of the muscle
   D. Is transmitted via A delta afferent and gamma efferent fibres
   E. Prevents tetanic oscillation between opposing muscle groups

QUESTION 41

The Rotameter

   A. Is a variable orifice flowmeter
   B. Is susceptible to static electricity
   C. Should be accurate to within 0.2%
   D. Consists of a bobbin in a parallel-sided tube
   E. The bobbin has vanes to help it to spin freely

QUESTION 42

Nitric oxide (NO)

   A. Is synthesised exclusively by vascular endothelium
   B. Is synthesised from L-asparagine in a process dependent on NO synthase
   C. Is produced by the normal human lung and is present in exhaled gas
   D. Binds to haemoglobin with an affinity equal to that of carbon monoxide (CO)
   E. Ultimately is metabolised to nitrate which is excreted by the kidneys

QUESTION 43

Acetazolamide

A. Increases the production of hydrogen ions by the renal tubule
B. Is used in the treatment of glaucoma
C. Can only be given orally
D. Causes the retention of chloride ions
E. Leads to a metabolic acidosis by enhancing the excretion of bicarbonate from the proximal tubule

QUESTION 44

The following are monoamine oxidase inhibitors

A. Phenelzine
B. Isocarboxazid
C. Paroxetine
D. Moclobemide
E. Fluoxetine

QUESTION 45

Concerning ranitidine

A. It has an imidazole structure
B. It enhances gastric emptying
C. About 50% is excreted unchanged by the kidney
D. It is more potent than cimetidine in antagonising hydrogen ion secretion by gastric parietal cells
E. It binds less avidly to cytochrome P_{450} than cimetidine

QUESTION 46

Recommended standards of monitoring

A. The most important monitor is the pulse oximeter
B. It is not necessary to have a capnograph
C. Blood pressure measurement is only required for operations of over ten minutes duration
D. Only an ECG and non-invasive blood pressure are required for regional anaesthesia
E. The main cause of anaesthetic mortality is equipment failure

QUESTION 47

With regard to lithium carbonate

A. It equilibrates rapidly with the CSF
B. It is not reabsorbed from the glomerular filtrate by the renal tubule
C. It can lead to hyperthyroidism
D. The addition of thiazide diuretics can precipitate lithium toxicity
E. It can lead to ECG changes, including peaked T waves

QUESTION 48

Regarding the adverse effects of thiopentone

A. Hypersensitivity reactions occur with an approximate frequency of 1/1500
B. It is relatively contra-indicated in hepatic porphyria
C. It is associated with the development of laryngospasm
D. Erotic dreams are reported by patients following emergence from anaesthesia with thiopentone
E. A 2.5% solution is used to abolish sequelae of accidental intra-arterial injection

QUESTION 49

Concerning renal disease

A. Gallamine is a useful non-depolarising neuromuscular blocker
B. It may present with haematuria
C. EDTA clearance can be used to quantify the extent of the impairment
D. Volatile anaesthetic agents are safe
E. Arterio-venous shunt formation can be carried out under regional anaesthesia

QUESTION 50

The following agents may be used safely in a patient with asthma

A. Vecuronium
B. Ketamine
C. Atracurium
D. Tubocurarine
E. Isoflurane

QUESTION 51

Comparing lignocaine with bupivacaine

A. Lignocaine has a higher pKa
B. Lignocaine is more extensively protein bound
C. Lignocaine is more potent
D. Lignocaine has a lower molecular weight
E. Lignocaine is less lipid soluble

QUESTION 52

Inguinal hernia field block

A. Blocks the ilioinguinal, iliohypogastric and genitofemoral nerves
B. May be employed for testicular surgery
C. Prilocaine 0.5% may be used
D. Depends on depositing local anaesthetic between internal and external oblique
E. Quadriceps weakness is a complication

QUESTION 53

Cystic fibrosis

A. Is an autosomal dominant condition with an incidence of 1:2000 live births
B. May present with meconium ileus
C. An anticholinergic is an essential part of premedication in order to reduce the incidence of bradycardia
D. Chest infection and cardiac failure are the usual mode of death from the condition in the adult
E. A low $PaCO_2$ is usual

QUESTION 54

Humidity is measured by

A. Measuring the elasticity of a rubber strip
B. Measuring the difference between the temperature of a dry thermometer and one kept wet
C. Measuring the change in the length of a hair
D. Assessing the temperature at which condensation occurs
E. Assessing electrical conductivity across an air gap

QUESTION 55

Inhalational anaesthetic agent concentration may be monitored clinically by

A. Measuring the change in elasticity of silicone rubber strips
B. Measuring the frequency of quartz crystal oscillation
C. Infra-red absorption analysis
D. Ultra-violet absorption analysis
E. Paramagnetic analysis

QUESTION 56

Carbamazepine

A. Induces hepatic microsomal enzymes
B. Often causes blood dyscrasias
C. Causes a rash in 10-20% of patients
D. Inhibits the metabolism of phenytoin
E. Can induce pancreatitis

QUESTION 57

Premedication

A. Sedation with lorazepam 2 mg is appropriate for an adult male
B. Oral atropine 20 mcg/kg is appropriate for a 4 year old child
C. The last dose of antihypertensive medication should be given the night before surgery
D. Tricyclic antidepressants must be discontinued two weeks prior to surgery
E. Ranitidine 150 mg and 0.3M sodium citrate 30 ml are components of obstetric premedication

QUESTION 58

The following are examples of phase II (conjugation) reactions

A. Glucuronidation
B. Oxidation
C. Methylation
D. Sulphation
E. Hydration

QUESTION 59

Concerning types of data

A. Blood pressures arranged in order represent ordinal data
B. Pain scores would be ordinal data
C. Survival and non-survival are nominal data
D. Femoral length is a discrete variable
E. Numbers of delivered DC shocks would be continuous variables

QUESTION 60

In the lung apex

A. $PaCO_2$ is higher than in basal alveoli
B. PcO_2 is higher than in basal capillaries
C. Capillary blood flow is greater than that in basal capillaries
D. Alveolar minute volume is less than that of basal alveoli
E. V/Q ratio remains approximately the same as in the lung base

QUESTION 61

During blood gas analysis

A. pH is derived from measured PCO_2
B. PO_2 is measured using a Clark electrode
C. PCO_2 is measured indirectly
D. Base excess is measured directly
E. Standard bicarbonate is derived rather than directly measured

QUESTION 62

Estimation of left ventricular preload using the assumption that the PCWP=LVEDP=LVEDV is inaccurate in the following settings

A. Mitral stenosis
B. Positive end expiratory pressure (PEEP)
C. Pulmonary artery catheter placed in West zone 3
D. Left atrial myxoma
E. Pulmonary stenosis

QUESTION 63

Venous air embolism

A. Is commoner in the sitting position than supine at craniotomy
B. Presents with a sudden onset
C. May be detected early by ECG changes
D. Trend display of end-tidal CO_2 is not reliable
E. The embolism may be retrieved by aspiration through a central venous cannula

QUESTION 64

Aldosterone

A. Plasma levels increase with standing
B. Production decreases with a fall in blood volume
C. Production decreases with a rise in plasma renin level
D. Increases urinary potassium excretion
E. May be produced by tumours of the adrenal cortex

QUESTION 65

In dental anaesthesia

A. Infection is a relative indication for general anaesthesia
B. Prophylactic antibiotics are often required in children with Down's syndrome
C. Nasal intubation is usual for inpatient dental surgery
D. A maxillary nerve block affects the third division of the trigeminal nerve
E. Adrenaline 1:80,000 may produce symptoms of toxicity

QUESTION 66

Dangers from humidifiers include

A. Scalding
B. Pseudomonas infection
C. Airway obstruction
D. Water overload
E. Hypothermia

QUESTION 67

The following can be used for gaseous oxygen analysis

A. Paramagnetism
B. Raman scattering
C. A galvanic (or fuel) cell
D. Mass spectrometry
E. Ultra-violet absorption spectroscopy

QUESTION 68

Confidence intervals

A. Are normally defined with p values of +/- 0.05
B. Relate data derived from a sample to the population from which that sample was drawn
C. Are wide if the sample size is small
D. Are wide if the variance of the population is large
E. The 95% confidence intervals for a value are calculated as +/-1.96 SEM from that value

QUESTION 69

Prolactin

A. Stimulates release of dopamine in the hypothalamus
B. Release is increased by suckling
C. Release is inhibited by TRH
D. Release is facilitated by morphine
E. Stimulates an increased release of FSH and LHRH

QUESTION 70

Concerning sleep

A. REM sleep is divided into four stages
B. REM sleep makes up 60% of total sleep time
C. REM sleep is associated with slow irregular low-amplitude waves on the EEG
D. NREM sleep is associated with tachypnoea
E. REM sleep is associated with penile erections

QUESTION 71

CO_2 transport in venous blood

A. Occurs predominantly by conversion to bicarbonate
B. Results in an increase in erythrocyte volume
C. Causes an efflux of hydrogen ions from the erythrocyte
D. Is inhibited by deoxygenation of haemoglobin
E. Can occur by carbamino bonding in plasma

QUESTION 72

Low dose aspirin therapy (75-150 mg/day)

A. Is effective in the secondary prevention of transient ischaemic attack and stroke

B. Reversibly inhibits the action of cyclo-oxygenase

C. Selectively inhibits platelet cyclo-oxygenase preserving vessel cyclo-oxygenase

D. Inhibits platelet function for up to two days following its cessation

E. Is associated with fewer adverse reactions than anticoagulants when used for TIA prophylaxis

QUESTION 73

Concerning sensory receptors

A. Meissners corpuscles are associated with proprioception

B. Ruffini corpuscles are associated with proprioception

C. Pacinian corpuscles are associated with proprioception

D. Free nerve endings are associated with nociception

E. Pacinian corpuscles are associated with touch

QUESTION 74

FRC can be measured using

A. Body plethysmography

B. Spirometry

C. Intra-oesophageal balloon

D. Nitrogen wash-out

E. Helium wash-in

QUESTION 75

The following ECG changes occur with hypokalaemia

A. Tall T waves

B. ST elevation

C. Loss of P waves

D. T wave inversion

E. Prominent U waves

QUESTION 76

The following are true

A. Disinfection must be preceded by decontamination

B. Sterilisation must be preceded by disinfection

C. Pasteurisation is a method of sterilisation

D. Hot steam sterilisation requires temperatures of 100°C or over

E. Dry heat alone is ineffective for sterilisation

QUESTION 77

Progesterone

A. Delays gastric emptying
B. Stimulates ventilation
C. Increases SVR
D. Levels take 6 weeks post-delivery to return to pre-pregnant values
E. Is thermogenic

QUESTION 78

The following pharmacological definitions are correct

A. A ligand is a molecule that interacts with a receptor
B. Tachyphylaxis is a type 1 immediate hypersensitivity reaction
C. Positive co-operativity means receptor occupancy at low concentrations increases apparent receptor affinity at higher concentrations
D. Volume of distribution is the plasma volume into which the drug is administered
E. At steady state, infusion rate equals elimination rate

QUESTION 79

In respiratory failure

A. The anion gap is invariably increased
B. The arterial PO_2 at rest, sea level and breathing air, in the absence of cardiac shunting, should be < 8 kPa
C. If accompanied by hypercapnea is referred to as type 2 respiratory failure
D. If due to intrapulmonary shunting may be rapidly corrected by adminstration of 100% oxygen
E. May be caused by increased metabolic demand

QUESTION 80

Ketamine

A. Is available as a racaemic mixture containing equal mixtures of two optical isomers
B. The isomers have the same pharmacological properties
C. Is highly protein bound
D. Is highly lipid soluble
E. Is metabolised in the liver in a process involving cytochrome P_{450}

QUESTION 81

In descriptive statistics

A. The mean is the sum of all measurements divided by the number in the group
B. The mean and the median are separated by the standard error of the mean
C. The mode is the most commonly observed subject
D. A Gaussian distribution is a normal distribution
E. Population and sample are the same thing

QUESTION 82

Concerning propofol

A. About 5% is excreted unchanged
B. The principal metabolite is propofol glucuronide
C. One of the metabolites causes a green discolouration of urine
D. A fat overload syndrome can follow prolonged infusions
E. The clearance exceeds hepatic blood flow

QUESTION 83

In the normal population

A. 1% of individuals will have already developed Rh antibodies
B. Transfusion of ABO compatible blood is associated with a 20% risk of incompatibility
C. Rhesus negativity is determined by the absence of the D antigen
D. Approximately 50% of subjects will not possess A or B antibodies
E. ABO incompatible red cells are destroyed by complement mediated lysis following binding of IgM antibodies

QUESTION 84

The following are side-effects of amiodarone

A. Hyperthyroidism
B. Tremor
C. Peripheral neuropathy
D. Lupus-like syndrome
E. Pleural effusions

QUESTION 85

Concerning transdermal drug administration

A. First-pass metabolism is avoided
B. Uptake will depend on skin thickness and temperature
C. Passage across subcutaneous fat is the rate limiting step in drug uptake
D. Suitable drugs include hyoscine, nitroglycerine and clonidine
E. Fentanyl and morphine have similar rates of transfer

QUESTION 86

Bile secretion is stimulated by

A. Increased hepatic blood flow
B. Vagal stimulation
C. Hypercholesterolaemia
D. An elevated level of bile salts in the blood
E. Insulin

QUESTION 87

The following increase the movement of fluid out of capillaries

A. Arteriolar vasoconstriction
B. Venous hypertension
C. Hypotension
D. Decrease in oncotic pressure
E. Decrease in hydrostatic pressure in capillaries

QUESTION 88

During the process of haemostasis

A. The extrinsic cascade is initiated by contact between factor XII and collagen fibres.
B. Vitamin K is required for the formation of prothrombin
C. Local vasoconstriction occurs in response to serotonin released by platelets
D. Antithrombin 3 induced release of oxalate from the endothelium prevents extension of the clot
E. Enteral administration of antibiotics may affect clotting

QUESTION 89

The Coroner must be informed

A. If the patient died following surgery
B. When a patient who was receiving a war pension dies
C. If the patient was only seen by a doctor ten days prior to death
D. Following a fatal road traffic accident
E. If death occurred following paracetamol overdose

QUESTION 90

An increase in pulse pressure occurs

A. With a decrease in systemic vascular resistance
B. When measured in the foot as opposed to the forearm
C. With decreased myocardial contractility
D. In the elderly
E. On assuming the upright position from supine

Exam 5: Answers

ANSWER 1

A. FALSE   B. TRUE   C. FALSE   D. FALSE   E. TRUE

Nerve endings take up L-tyrosine. Synthesis to noradrenaline is rate-limited by the step converting tyrosine to L-Dopa, which is subject to negative feedback by noradrenaline. Presynaptic alpha 2 receptors exert a negative influence on release of presynaptic vesicles. Once released, termination of NA action occurs by diffusion into capillaries, presynaptic reuptake and subsequent inactivation by MAO, or extraneuronal uptake and inactivation by intracellular COMT.

Ref: Despopoulos A, Silbernagl S. Color Atlas of Physiology, 50-59

ANSWER 2

A. TRUE   B. FALSE   C. TRUE   D. TRUE   E. TRUE

Most iron in plasma is found as transferrin but there are small amounts of ferritin in plasma. 70% of whole body iron is in haemoglobin. In iron deficiency total transferrin concentrations are raised but saturation is reduced.

Ref: Ganong WF. Review of Medical Physiology, Lange

ANSWER 3

A. TRUE   B. FALSE   C. FALSE   D. FALSE   E. TRUE

Kwashiorkor is common in the tropics amongst those living on a diet adequate in calories, but grossly deficient in animal protein. The essential amino acids are required to maintain normal growth and nitrogen balance. In deficiency urea & uric acid excretion fall. Creatinine excretion is not affected. Urea nitrogen excretion will drop to c. 2.2 g/day. Anaemia and a fatty enlarged liver may occur.

Ref: Ganong WF. Review of Medical Physiology. Lange, Ch17

ANSWER 4

A. TRUE   B. TRUE   C. TRUE   D. FALSE   E. TRUE

Simple liquid-in-glass thermometers are cheap and in common use. The mercury thermometer has a wide range from its melting point (-39°C) up beyond 200°C. Electrical means of measuring temperature include:The resistance thermometer that relies on the linear change in the resistance of a platinum wire with temperature. It is not very sensitive and sensitivity is improved by use of a Wheatstone bridge configuration.The thermistor consists of a metal oxide bead that can be very small. This also changes its resistance with changing temperature, but in an exponential manner. It is much more sensitive in the clinical range. Its calibration is liable to change as it is subjected to major changes in temperature. Where two metals come into contact a current is produced, the voltage of which is dependant on the temperature of the junction (the Seebeck effect). Another junction is then connected into the circuit at a reference temperature. The voltage produced is linearly related to the temperature of the measuring junction.

Ref: Davis PD, Parbrook GD, Kenny GNC. Basic Physics and Measurement in Anaesthesia, 4th edn. Butterworth-Heinemann, 1995

ANSWER 5

A. FALSE   B. FALSE   C. TRUE   D. TRUE   E. TRUE

It binds to alpha-1 receptors selectively leaving alpha-2 mediated feedback on the release of noradrenaline intact. This accounts for the absence of reflex tachycardia. It does cause first dose hypotension particularly in those who are relatively fluid depleted and is thus highly unsuitable for the treatment of malignant hypertension where rapid falls in blood pressure are undesirable.

ANSWER 6

A. TRUE   B. TRUE   C. TRUE   D. TRUE   E. FALSE

Carotid sinus massage is manual stimulation of the carotid sinus baroreceptors, thus causing reflex inhibition of the vasomotor centre and stimulating the cardio-inhibitory centre. This results in bradycardia, and may restore sinus rhythm in patients with SVT. It reduces CBF by carotid artery compression and should therefore not be prolonged. Volatile anaesthetics abolish baroreceptor responses.

Ref: Yentis, Hirsch, Smith. Anaesthesia A to Z. Butterworth-Heinemann.

ANSWER 7

A. TRUE   B. FALSE   C. TRUE   D. FALSE   E. FALSE

It acts by interfering with the iodination of thyronines, a process requiring peroxidase. Small amounts are released in to the breast milk but provided the dose is low and fetal thyroid function is monitored its use in this setting is not contraindicated. Carbimazole is effective in inhibiting the formation of new and not stored hormone. Therefore it takes a few days before the clinical effects are seen and a few months before the patient is rendered euthyroid. Since it increases the vascularity of the gland it is usually replaced by a beta blocker and potassium iodide before surgery.

Ref: Sasada, Smith. Drugs in Anaesthesia and Intensive Care

ANSWER 8

A. FALSE   B. TRUE   C. FALSE   D. FALSE   E. TRUE

Ambient pressure doubles for every 10m depth in sea water and every 10.4m depth in fresh water. PO_2 increases proportionately. Air embolism is only possible if a breath was taken at depth. HPNS develops on deep dives using helium : oxygen mixes and gives rise to tremors, somnolence, and depressed A-wave activity on the EEG.

Ref: Ganong WF. Review of Medical Physiology. Lange, Ch37

ANSWER 9

A. FALSE   B. TRUE   C. TRUE   D. FALSE   E. FALSE

Most drugs metabolism occurs as a first order process (ie a constant proportion of the drug is metabolized in unit time). Alcohol metabolism is zero order (ie constant amount in unit time). Substances such as thiopentone and phenytoin have saturable elimination pathways such that metabolism is first order at low concentrations of the drug but zero order at high concentrations. As a result of this, the INCREASE in blood concentration may be higher than expected for a given top up dose if it is given when plasma concentrations are already elevated.

Ref: Nimmo, Rowbotham, Smith. Anaesthesia, Blackwell, chapter 15

ANSWER 10

A. TRUE · B. FALSE   C. FALSE   D. TRUE   E. FALSE

Any complex repeating waveform can be broken down into a fundamental and a number of harmonics. The more harmonics used, the closer to the original wave it is possible to get. Fourier analysis is this process.

Boyle's Law states that $P \times V$ = constant, or that $P = k/V$, and so the graph seen is a rectangular hyperbola.

Exponential functions are common in medicine. The commonest is the exponential decay function (pressure change as the oxygen within a cylinder escapes is an example of this). In this $P = P_0 . e^{(-kt)}$ as the value of P falls as time increases. An exponential function can be linearised by log transformation (with a slope of k or -k). The characteristics of the exponential decay function can be described either by the half-life or by the time constant (greek letter tau) which equals $1/k$. The time constant is considered to be the time taken to reach zero if the initial rate of fall were continued, or the time taken to reach 0.368 (= $1/e$) of the original value.

Ref: Sykes MK, Vickers MD, Hull CJ. Principles of Measurement and Monitoring in Anaesthesia and Intensive Care, 3rd edn. Blackwell Scientific Publishers, 1991

ANSWER 11

A. TRUE   B. FALSE   C. TRUE   D. TRUE   E. TRUE

2,3-DPG is formed in red blood cells from phosphoglyceraldehyde, a product of glycolysis. It binds strongly to the beta chains of haemoglobin (hence fetal haemoglobin has a low affinity) reducing oxygen binding and shifting the O2 dissociation curve to the right, thus favouring oxygen liberation to the tissues. Its concentration is increased by increased circulating thyroid hormones and growth hormone and androgens.

Ref: Ganong WF. Review of Medical Physiology. Lange, Ch27.

ANSWER 12

A. TRUE   B. TRUE   C. FALSE   D. TRUE   E. FALSE

It may cause megaloblastic anaemia, aplastic anaemia, thrombocytopenia, leukopenia. Corneal deposits are a side effect of amiodarone. Other complications of phenytoin include hirsuitism, and gingival hyperplasia. Valproate causes gastric irritation. Other side effects: Nausea and vomiting, headache, dizziness, insomnia, confusion.

Ref: BNF1996

ANSWER 13

A. TRUE   B. TRUE   C. FALSE   D. FALSE   E. TRUE

The macrolides eg erythromycin inhibit mRNA translation; metronidazole inhibits mRNA transcription.

ANSWER 14

A. TRUE   B. FALSE   C. TRUE   D. FALSE   E. TRUE

When using a circle system the elimination of carbon dioxide depends on the passage of the expired gases through effective soda lime. Failure of the valves or inadvertent bypassing of the absorber will lead to carbon dioxide rebreathing. If the soda lime is not properly packed the gas may pass through low resistance channels, causing a local exhaustion of the soda lime, whilst the indicator on the outside looks good. Disconnection of the endotracheal tube should not lead to rebreathing (assuming there are no drapes restricting the free circulation of air around the open end of the tube). Similarly failure of the oxygen supply will lead to hypoxia but not to rebreathing of carbon dioxide.

Ref: Dorsch JA, Dorsch SE. Understanding Anesthesia Equipment; Construction, Care and Complications, 2nd edn. Wlliams & Wilkins, 1984

ANSWER 15

A. TRUE   B. TRUE   C. FALSE   D. FALSE   E. TRUE

All nephrons possess a loop of Henle, 20% will be juxtamedullary. Proximal tubular cells are particularly rich in mitochondria.

Ref: Despopoulos A, Silbernagl S. Color Atlas of Physiology. 120-150.

ANSWER 16

A. TRUE   B. TRUE   C. TRUE   D. FALSE   E. TRUE

Tricyclic antidepressants potentiate the action of endogenous amines in the brain. They also exhibit anti-muscarinic, histaminergic and adrenergic effects. They exhibit a wide range of cardiovascular, neurological and autonomic side effects. Postural hypotension, tachydysrhythmias, and increased P-R and Q-T intervals can all occur. Respiratory depression and sedation are possible. Anticholinergic effects include blurred vision, dry mouth, constipation and urinary retention. The cardiovascular effects of direct and indirect acting sympathomimetics may be potentiated.

Ref: Sasada, Smith. Drugs in Anaesthesia and Intensive Care

ANSWER 17

A. FALSE   B. FALSE   C. TRUE   D. FALSE   E. FALSE

Parametric tests are used in the analysis of normally distributed data. Student's t-test compares the mean and SD for two groups. Cochrane's test is a non parametric test applied to more than two groups of nominal data. Fisher's exact test is substituted for the Chi squared test if the expected frequency is less than 5. Spearman's rank correlation test ranks ordinal non parametric data. Spearman's correlation is however a parametric test comparing two variables for association. Weber's test is a clinical test for deafness!!!

Ref: Yentis, Hirsch, Smith. Anaesthesia A to Z. Butterworth-Heinemann

ANSWER 18

A. FALSE   **B. FALSE**   **C. TRUE**   **D. TRUE**   **E. TRUE**

Flow = [Pressure difference x Pi x (fourth power of radius)] / [8 x length x VISCOSITY]. Also don't forget that Flow = Pressure difference/RESISTANCE. Blood viscosity depends on haematocrit. If the radius of a vessel is doubled, resistance will fall to 6% of its previous value.

Ref: Ganong WF. Review of Medical Physiology. Lange, Ch30

ANSWER 19

A. TRUE   **B. FALSE**   **C. TRUE**   **D. TRUE**   **E. FALSE**

The angiotensin converting enzyme inhibitors have an anti-aldosterone effect They act as weak potassium sparing diuretics and concomittant use of such drugs should be undertaken with care.

Ref: BNF 1996

ANSWER 20

A. TRUE   **B. TRUE**   **C. FALSE**   **D. TRUE**   **E. FALSE**

Three things are needed for a fire to occur: a source of fuel, an oxidising agent (not necessarily oxygen or air) and some form of energy to activate the process (not necessarily heat)

Ref: Davis PD, Parbrook GD, Kenny GNC. Basic Physics and Measurement in Anaesthesia, 4th edn. Butterworth-Heinemann, 1995

ANSWER 21

A. TRUE   **B. FALSE**   **C. TRUE**   **D. TRUE**   **E. FALSE**

Dopamine is a precursor of adrenaline. Dobutamine is a synthetic compound. The synthetic pathway is as follows:

Tyrosine-DOPA-Dopamine-Noradrenaline-Adrenaline

Ref: Aitkenhead, Smith. Textbook of Anaesthesia. Churchill Livingstone

ANSWER 22

A. FALSE   **B. TRUE**   **C. TRUE**   **D. FALSE**   **E. TRUE**

The murmur of aortic stenosis should be investigated to establish the degree of stenosis and the gradient across the valve, as a fixed-output state has implications for the safety of procedures such as regional block and in any situation where systemic vascular resistance may alter. The Royal College of Radiologists (1979) state that CXR is justified where there is acute respiratory distress, metastatic disease, pulmonary TB and in chronic airways disease with no recent CXR; it is fairly unhelpful in CCF, where clinical signs are more instructive. Low serum potassium is a frequent finding in the presence of a diuretic and is important because of the risk of tachyarrhythmia under anaesthesia. A single ECG in isolation will identify less than a quarter of those patients with ischaemic heart disease; exercise ECG may be helpful, and the comparison with previous ECG recordings may demonstrate a change indicating an ischaemic event in the interval between recordings; however a single ECG recording cannot be regarded as a sensitive investigation. Haemoglobin measurement in young people is generally unhelpful but is justified in menstruating women because of the (remote) possibility of anaemia.

ANSWER   23

A. FALSE   B. FALSE   C. FALSE   D. FALSE   E. FALSE

Its analgesic potency is one fifth to one tenth that of morphine. It also has actions on alpha-2 receptors (antagonised by yohimbine), noradrenaline & 5HT reuptake. It has an inactive metabolite. Theoretically should not be used in patients on monoamine oxidase inhibitors because of its effects on the activation of noradrenergic pathways.

Ref: British Journal of Anaesthesia 1995; 74(3): 247 (Editorial)

Drugs and Therapeutics Bulletin 1994; 32: 11

ANSWER   24

A. TRUE   B. TRUE   C. FALSE   D. FALSE   E. FALSE

TIVA is implicated in many cases of awareness especially in the paralysed patient. It is not reported when adequate amounts of volatile agent are used, and the agent monitor, appropriately adjusted, is most useful; the default setting is the factory-preset alarm limit, and is usually 0% for the low alarm level, which is of course no use in this respect and has to be adjusted for it to be meaningful. The PRST score is blood pressure, heart rate, sweat and tears scored 0-2 for each; a score of 4 is said to indicate surgical anaesthesia. The BSI ranges from 0 (dead) to 100 (awake) but coma may score 50 and be unrousable whereas natural sleep may score 20 and be immediately rousable. Midazolam has no retrograde amnesic effects.

ANSWER   25

A. FALSE   B. TRUE   C. FALSE   D. FALSE   E. TRUE

Plots log PCO_2 against pH. After measuring the original pH of the sample a CO_2 titration line is constructed by equilibrating the sample with 2 gases of known PCO_2. pH is remeasured in each case allowing the original PCO_2 to be read against its pH. PCO_2 is never measured. Standard bicarbonate is extrapolated from a secondary x-axis that intersects the y-axis at normal PCO_2. Base excess and buffer base content (Protein, HCO_3, Hb) are estimated from intersections with two curved scales.

Ref: Ganong WF. Review of Medical Physiology. Lange, Ch40

ANSWER   26

A. FALSE   B. FALSE   C. TRUE   D. FALSE   E. FALSE

A fluid is a substance that cannot sustain a shearing force. It includes liquids gases and vapours. The gaseous phase is defined as that in which a substance expands to occupy the space in which it is confined. A vapour is a substance in the gaseous phase at or below its critical temperature.

Heat is energy; temperature represents the average kinetic energy of a substance. This is reduced to zero as the molecular movement slows and then stops at absolute zero. 1 calorie is the energy required to raise 1 gram of water through from 14.5 to 15.5°C at 1 atm.

Ref: Urquhart JC, Blunt MC. The Anaesthesia Viva: Physiology, Pharmacology and Statistics, Greenwich Medical Media, 1996

ANSWER 27

A. TRUE   B. FALSE   C. FALSE   D. TRUE   E. TRUE

Vomiting causes loss of hydrogen, sodium, potassium and chloride ions. Subsequent alkalosis leads to renal bicarbonate loss and alkaline urine. However, as the sodium falls increased aldosterone production leads to renal sodium and water retention at the expense of potassium and hydrogen ions. If the ensuing hypokalaemia becomes profound the kidneys will secrete hydrogen ions in order to conserve potassium, leading to paradoxical acid urine.

Ref: Ganong WF. Review of Medical Physiology. Lange.

ANSWER 28

A. FALSE   B. FALSE   C. TRUE   D. FALSE   E. TRUE

Hypermagnesaemia is rare but may become more important as magnesium is used increasingly in therapy eg for eclampsia. It tends to act as a vasodilator and can cause hypotension, delayed cardiac conduction, nausea and vomiting, muscle weakness with hyporeflexia and ultimately respiratory impairment, hence hypercapnia. Tetany occurs with hypomagnesaemia and more commonly with hypocalcaemia.

Ref: Yentis, Hirsch, Smith. Anaesthesia A to Z. Butterworth-Heinemann

ANSWER 29

A. TRUE   B. TRUE   C. FALSE   D. FALSE   E. TRUE

IgM does exist as a pentamer and is principally involved with complement fixation. IgA is secretory and appears in breast milk along with other secretions. IgG crosses the placenta and IgE is involved in mast cell degranulation.

Ref: Ganong WF. Review of Medical Physiology. Lange. Ch27.

ANSWER 30

A. FALSE   B. TRUE   C. TRUE   D. TRUE   E. TRUE

GABA is an inhibitory mediator in the brain and retina, responsible for pre-synaptic inhibition. It is formed by the decarboxylation of glutamate and functions by increasing chloride ion conductance, an effect which is enhanced by the benzodiazepines giving them sedative properties.

Ref: Ganong WF. Review of Medical Physiology. Lange.

ANSWER 31

A. FALSE   B. TRUE   C. FALSE   D. TRUE   E. TRUE

The mechanism of its action has still to be fully elucidated: it does antagonise adenosine receptors but it is doubtful whether this is the mechanism for the production of bronchodilation. The inhibition of phosphodiesterase with reductions in intracellular calcium is still firm favourite as chief mechanism. It is a CNS stimulant.

Ref: Kaufmann, Taberner. Pharmacology in the Practice of Anaesthesia. Arnold, Chapter 19, part II

ANSWER 32

A. FALSE   B. FALSE   C. TRUE   D. TRUE   E. FALSE

It is manufactured by the thermal decomposition of ammonium nitrate (!). It causes a rise in PVR especially in patients with pre-existing pulmonary hypertension and causes a rise in sympathetic outflow. It inhibits methionine synthetase by irreversibly oxidising vitamin B_{12} from the active cob(I)alamin to the inactive cob(III)alamin. As cob(I)alamin is a co-enzyme for methionine synthetase, the oxidation of vit B_{12} effectively inactivates the enzyme. The enzyme is essential in folate and thymidine metabolism and the result is megaloblastic bone marrow changes and subacute combined degeneration of the cord.

Ref: Current Anaesthesia and Intensive Care 1994; 5: 109-114

ANSWER 33

A. TRUE   B. TRUE   C. TRUE   D. FALSE   E. FALSE

There is a higher incidence of allergic reactions than with the gelatins and this may be associated with antibodies to recent pneumococcal infections. Both Dextran 70 and 40 may interfere with cross-matching. They can form a complex with fibrinogen and so induce a coagulopathy. This may be useful in the prophylaxis of venous thromboembolism. The currently used ones have an average molecular weight of 40 or 70 kDa.

ANSWER 34

A. TRUE   B. TRUE   C. FALSE   D. FALSE   E. TRUE

It contains an ester linkage which, when cleaved, yields the acid metabolite. A basic drug, existing at a pH above its pKa will be largely unionized and therefore more lipid soluble. This property, unlike fentanyl which is 90% ionised at body pH, accounts for its rapid onset of action. It is largely broken down by tissue (probably skeletal muscle) esterases. The half life of remifentanil in whole blood is 65 minutes. This is not affected by neostigmine and the drug is not affected by pseudocholinesterase. Remifentanil does not accumulate, its rapid hydrolysis accounts for its short duration of action.

Ref: Seminars in Anesthesia 1996; 15(1)

ANSWER 35

A. FALSE   B. TRUE   C. FALSE   D. FALSE   E. FALSE

The Manley ventilator is still the commonest ventiltor in use in the UK despite its age. It is neither a flow generator nor a true pressure generator, though its function is similar to the latter. It is a minute volume divider. It is normally used without a circle system, but like all ventilators must be fitted with a disconnection device. It contains two bellows and three valves.

ANSWER 36

A. TRUE   B. FALSE   C. FALSE   D. TRUE   E. TRUE

A capacitor may be thought of as two conductors separated by an insulator. It is able to store charge (not CURRENT which is charge flow per unit time), and is therefore the basis of the defibrillator. It has a resistance to current flow that consists of two components, one that is simple resistance and a second that is inversely proportional to a.c. frequency (reactance). Capacitance is measured in Farads (1 Farad = 1 Coulomb per Volt).

Ref: Strickland DAP. Physical principles. In: Scurr C, Feldman S, Soni N (Eds) Scientific Foundations of Anaesthesia; The Basis of Intensive Care, 4th edn. Heinemann Medical Books, 1990, pp 10-51

ANSWER 37

A. TRUE   B. TRUE   C. TRUE   D. FALSE   E. FALSE

Mannitol increases intravascular fluid volume via its effect on plasma osmolarity, and may precipitate pulmonary oedema. It is used to treat raised intra-cranial pressure in fulminant hepatic failure and the hepato-renal syndrome. Mannitol does not cross the blood-brain barrier. The usual dose is 0.25-1g/kg.

PHYSICAL:

10% = 550 mOsm/kg, 20% = 1100 mOsm/kg

Ref: Yentis, Hirsch, Smith. Anaesthesia A to Z . Butterworth-Heinemann

ANSWER 38

A. FALSE   B. FALSE   C. TRUE   D. FALSE   E. TRUE

Captopril competitively inhibits angiotensin I converting enzyme, preventing the conversion of angiotensin I to angiotensin II. Angiotensin II stimulates the secretion of aldosterone by the adrenal cortex. Thus captopril causes a decrease in plasma angiotensin II and aldosterone, and an increase in renin levels. About 25% is reversibly protein bound, and about 50% is excreted unchanged. Enalapril can be given once daily. Captopril can cause thrombocytopenia, neutropenia and agranulocytosis.

ANSWER 39

A. FALSE   B. TRUE   C. FALSE   D. TRUE   E. TRUE

Stimulation of vagal fibres to the heart dilates the coronaries, flow is reduced but continues through ventricular systole in the right coronary, but not in the left. Local vasodilator metabolites active in the coronaries include potassium and adenosine (cf skeletal muscle.) Coronary blood flow can be measured using a variation of the Kety method.

Ref: Ganong WF. Review of Medical Physiology. Lange. Ch32.

ANSWER 40

A. FALSE   B. TRUE   C. TRUE   D. FALSE   E. FALSE

When muscle tension exceeds a certain threshold, relaxation occurs in response to strong stretch detected by Golgi tendon organs located in series with muscle fibres. Ib myelinated afferents produce IPSPs on motor neurones, and excitatory connections with antagonistic muscle motor neurones.

Ref: Ganong WF. Review of Medical Physiology. Lange, Ch6

ANSWER 41

A. TRUE   B. TRUE   C. FALSE   D. FALSE   E. TRUE

The Rotameter is a variable orifice (as opposed to fixed orifice) flowmeter. It contains a bobbin with vanes that help it spin and so reduce the effect of friction between the wall of the tube and the bobbin itself. The tube is conical and it is the changing size of the annular orifice around the constantly-sized bobbin as it rises up the tube that provides the variable orifice. An accurately calibrated and mounted Rotameter may be accurate to within 2%. It is susceptible to static electricity which is why there is a internal coating of a transparent layer of tin oxide on the tube to conduct the static charge away to earth. If you knew this and reasoned that the Rotameter is therefore resistant to static charge and so answered 'false' then you should realise that a number of questions in the exam may be ambiguous and that this may be a question to leave blank

Ref: Mushin WM, Jones PL. Physics for the Anaesthetist, 4th edn. Blackwell Scientific Publications, 1987

ANSWER 42

A. FALSE   B. FALSE   C. TRUE   D. FALSE   E. TRUE

Nitric oxide is also produced by macrophages and thrombocytes. There are two types of NO synthase, a calcium dependent and a calcium independent form. It is synthesised from L-arginine. The haemoglobin molecule has an affinity 1500 times higher to NO than to CO. Nitrosyl haemoglobin is produced, which in the presence of oxygen, is oxidised to methaemoglobin. Nitrate is ultimately produced after regeneration of haemoglobin by methaemoglobin reductase in red blood cells. Inhaled NO improves oxygenation in patients with ARDS by pulmonary vasodilatation in areas of ventilated alveoli, thus diverting blood flow away from areas of intrapulmonary shunt to areas of more normal V/Q ratio. NO is rapidly de-activated in blood and systemic hypotension does not occur. Conversely, following the use of systemically applied vasodilators such as prostacyclin and sodium nitroprusside, there may be an increase in shunt and a fall in systemic pressure and oxygen tension.

Ref: British Journal of Anaesthesia 1995; 74: 443

ANSWER 43

A. FALSE   B. TRUE   C. FALSE   D. TRUE   E. FALSE

Acetazolamide inhibits carbonic anhydrase, thereby diminishing hydrogen ion production in the renal tubules. Increased bicarbonate ion excretion takes place in the distal tubule. It may be given orally and intravenously for the acute reduction in intraocular pressure. It is also used in the treatment of mountain sickness.

ANSWER 44

A. TRUE   B. TRUE   C. FALSE   D. TRUE   E. FALSE

Paroxetine and fluoxetine are selective serotonin re-uptake inhibitors (SSRIs). They are effective antidepressants, and are less sedative than the tricyclics.

Ref: BNF 1996

ANSWER 45

A. FALSE   B. FALSE   C. TRUE   D. TRUE   E. TRUE

Ranitidine has a furan ring, unlike cimetidine which has an imidazole ring. It does not affect gastric emptying or lower oesophageal sphincter tone. It does not have the same antiandrogenic, antidopaminergic or cytochrome P_{450} mediated metabolism that is associated with cimetidine.

PHYSICAL:

15% protein bound, Vd 1.2-1.8 l/kg, bio-availability 50-60%

DOSE:

50 mg 8 hrly orally, 150 mg slow iv 12 hrly

Ref: Sasada, Smith. Drugs in Anaesthesia & Intensive Care

ANSWER 46

A. FALSE   B. FALSE   C. FALSE   D. FALSE   E. FALSE

The main cause of anaesthetic mortality is human error. It was felt in the mid 1980s that improvement of the standards of monitoring would help reduce this. The first standard came from Harvard Medical School and this was rapidly adopted in the U.K. In 1988 the Association of Anaesthetists published its guidelines, which were updated in 1994. These are obligatory reading for anyone sitting Royal College examinations. The most fundamental and important monitor is THE CONTINUOUS PRESENCE OF THE ANAESTHETIST. This should be supplemented by an oxygen analyser, and it is strongly recommended that continuous ECG, pulse rate and volume and oxygen saturation be monitored. Blood pressure must be recorded regularly. A pulse oximeter and capnograph MUST be available for every patient. These recommendations (with others) apply to ALL anaesthetics, including regional and local anaesthesia as well as some cases in which sedation is used. Legally the guidelines are being seen as safe practice, and to ignore them may be seen as negligent.

Ref: Association of Anaesthetists Recommendations for Standards of Monitoring during Anaesthesia and Recovery. Revised edn. The Association of Anaesthetists of Great Britain and Ireland, 1994

ANSWER 47

A. FALSE   B. FALSE   C. FALSE   D. TRUE   E. FALSE

Lithium is used in the treatment of manic depression. Its use can lead to sodium retention and oedema, thyroid enlargement and hypothyroidism, polyuria and polydipsia, T wave depression, and enhanced responses to neuromuscular blockers. The therapeutic range is narrow. Addition of thiazides can cause lithium retention. Toxicity manifests as drowsiness, muscle weakness, dysrhythmias, hypotension and seizures. Passage across the blood brain barrier is slow and incomplete. 80% of filtered lithium is reabsorbed.

ANSWER 48

A. FALSE   B. FALSE   C. TRUE   D. TRUE   E. FALSE

Hypersensitivity reactions occur with a frequency one tenth or less of that quoted above! It is ABSOLUTELY contra-indicated in porphyria. Sadly, thiopentone does not lead to erotic dreams. The use of a 2.5% solution will reduce the incidence and severity of complications following an intra-arterial injection but will not remove the risk altogether.

ANSWER 49

A. FALSE   B. TRUE   C. FALSE   D. TRUE   E. TRUE

Renal disease may present with haematuria, proteinuria, hypertension or uraemia (or its symptoms). Gallamine is principally excreted renally and is a poor choice in renal disease. Safe anaesthetic include induction agents, atracurium, opiates and volatiles. EDTA clearance confirms normal function but does not quantify abnormality; PAH clearance is used for renal plasma flow, creatinine clearance for the glomerular filtration rate. Formation of shunt under local or regional anaesthesia is often a very good choice.

ANSWER   50

A. TRUE   B. TRUE   C. FALSE   D. FALSE   E. TRUE

Agents which provoke histamine release should be avoided because of risk of provoking bronchospasm which may be life threatening. These include atracurium, thiopentone and tubocurarine. Ketamine will cause bronchodilation, as do·volatile anaesthetic agents despite the respiratory irritant effects of isoflurane when used for the induction of anaesthesia. Non steroidals should be used with caution in patients know to have asthma.

ANSWER   51

A. FALSE   B. FALSE   C. FALSE   D. TRUE   E. TRUE

LIGNOCAINE

pKa = 7.9

MWt = 234

Partition coefficient = 2.9

Protein binding = 64%

Relative potency = 1

BUPIVACAINE pKa = 8.1

MWt = 288

Partition coefficient = 27.5

Protein binding = 96%

Relative potency = 4

Partition coefficient indicates lipid solubility and as a consequence, relates to potency.

Protein binding primarily influences duration of action.

pKa influences degree of ionization and therefore speed of onset.

Ref: Nunn, Utting, Brown. General Anaesthesia. Butterworths.

ANSWER   52

A. TRUE   B. FALSE   C. TRUE   D. TRUE   E. TRUE

Local anaesthetic is deposited between the internal and external oblique muscle layers. If the internal oblique is penetrated, local anaesthetic may track back to the lumbar plexus and affect the femoral nerve, producing quadriceps weakness. Prilocaine may be used because of the larger amount of solution which may safely be injected, but most would use bupivacaine. The testicle is innervated by T10 and so this block is quite ineffective for testicular surgery.

ANSWER   53

A. FALSE   B. TRUE   C. FALSE   D. TRUE   E. TRUE

Cystic fibrosis is an autosomal recessive condition with the gene carried by 1:25 of the population. It may present with meconium ileus or malabsorption, although it is the respiratory and cardiac manifestations of the condition which are of the greatest interest in anaesthesia. Recurrent infections lead to bronchiectasis and pulmonary fibrosis. Pulmonary hypertension and eventual right heart failure follow. With improved medical management, more of these patients are surviving to reach adulthood, when they present for transplantation. An anticholinergic is useful in paediatric anaesthesia, but if given as a premedicant will further reduce the viscosity of airway secretions and impair breathing. Better to give it at induction and use humidified gases. Hypoxaemia is common, and the $PaCO_2$ is low unless the lung disease is severe.

Ref: Walsh et al. Anaesthesia and cystic fibrosis. Anaesthesia 1995;50:614

ANSWER 54

A. FALSE   B. TRUE   C. TRUE   D. TRUE   E. FALSE

Three methods are used to measure humidity:

Hair hygrometer - measures the change in length of a hair.

Wet and dry bulb hygrometer - measures the difference in the temperature between a dry thermometer and a wet thermometer that occurs due to evaporation.

Regnault's hygrometer - measures the dew point on a test tube cooled by bubbling air through ether.

Rubber elasticity is used to measure anaesthetic agent concentration. Although electrical conductivity will change with humidity it is not used for measurement.

Ref: Davis PD, Parbrook GD, Kenny GNC. Basic Physics and Measurement in Anaesthesia, 4th edn. Butterworth-Heinemann, 1995

ANSWER 55

A. TRUE   B. TRUE   C. TRUE   D. TRUE   E. FALSE

There have been many methods for measuring anaesthetic agent concentration, with varying success, including the use of rubber strips (Drager narcotest), quartz crystals (Engström multi-gas monitor for anaesthesia; EMMA), ultra-violet absorption analysis for halothane, infra-red analysis and Raman scattering. Paramagnetic measurement is concerned with oxygen analysis.

Ref: Dorsch JA, Dorsch SE Understanding Anesthesia Equipment; Construction, Care and Complications, 2nd edn. Wlliams & Wilkins, 1984

ANSWER 56

A. TRUE   B. FALSE   C. TRUE   D. TRUE   E. FALSE

Blood dyscrasias are very rare; more common with the use of sodium valproate. Pancreatitis is also a side effect of valproate.

Ref: Drugs and Therapeutics Bulletin 1994; 32(6): 45

ANSWER 57

A. TRUE   B. TRUE   C. FALSE   D. FALSE   E. TRUE

The risk from tricyclic medication is from direct acting vasopressors such as adrenaline, as these drugs block reuptake. They are also arrhythmogenic and vagolytic. Monoamine oxidase inhibitors prevent breakdown of catecholamines and the risk is from indirect acting vasopressors such as ephedrine. The standard teaching is that MAOI should be terminated at least 2 weeks before anaesthesia but this is frequently disregarded.

Anticholinergics are given to children to prevent excess secretions but also because of the vagal-dominance of this age group and the tendency to bradycardia. Most medication, including all cardiac and antihypertensive medication, should be continued up to and including the morning of surgery.

ANSWER 58

A. TRUE   B. FALSE   C. TRUE   D. TRUE   E. FALSE

Oxidation and hydration are examples of phase I reactions. Phase I & II reactions do not however have to occur in that order.

Ref: Kaufman, Taberner. Pharmacology in the Practice of Anaesthesia, Arnold, Chapter 3

ANSWER 59

A. FALSE   B. TRUE   C. TRUE   D. FALSE   E. FALSE

Femoral length is continuous because fractions of units of measurement apply, whereas only whole numbers of DC shocks can exist. Length and pressure are interval scale data. A pain score of 8 does not necessarily indicate pain twice as severe as represented by a score of 4; the score only serves to put the degree of pain in an order, and is therefore ordinal data.

ANSWER 60

A. FALSE   B. TRUE   C. FALSE   D. TRUE   E. FALSE

$PaCO_2$ rises from apex to base whereas $PaCO_2$ falls. $PcCO_2$ and PcO_2 levels show a similar trend. Alveolar minute volume rises from apex to base by a factor of x4 due to differences in the resting state of expansion and therefore compliance of the alveoli in each lung area. V/Q ratio is approximately x5 greater in the apex. Regional differences in perfusion are greater than regional differences in ventilation.

Ref: Despopoulos A, Silbernagl S. Color Atlas of Physiology, 78-108

ANSWER 61

A. FALSE   B. TRUE   C. TRUE   D. FALSE   E. TRUE

Blood gas analysers measure pH (glass electrode), PO_2 (Clark electrode), and conductance (Hb estimation). Everything else is derived. pH is measured before and after equilibration of the sample with reference gases of known PCO_2. A PCO_2 that corresponds to the original pH may thus be calculated.

ANSWER 62

A. TRUE   B. TRUE   C. FALSE   D. TRUE   E. FALSE

Left ventricular function relates in part to the myofibril length before contraction (estimated by left ventricular end-diastolic volume - LVEDV). If the compliance of the heart is normal this volume is in a proportional relationship with left ventricular end-diastolic pressure (LVEDP). Pulmonary capillary wedge pressure (PCWP) equates to LVEDP providing there is nothing interfering with pressure transmission between the left ventricle and the end of the pulmonary artery where the catheter is placed. Thus mitral valvular disease, left atrial myxoma and PEEP affect the relationship. The catheter should be placed in West zone 3 as in the upper lung fields (zones 1 and 2) the pulmonary veins collapse for all or part of the respiratory cycle.

Ref: Faust RJ (ed) Anesthesiology Review, 2nd edn. Churchill Livingstone, 1994

ANSWER   63

A. TRUE   B. FALSE   C. FALSE   D. FALSE   E. TRUE

The sitting position is rarely used in current practice for the very good reason that it was associated with a 45% incidence of venous air embolism. This is characteristically of insidious onset. However an acute bolus of 100 ml would be fatal in an adult. ECG changes occur late. Trend display of end-tidal CO_2, which would fall over a period of several minutes were an air embolism to be developing, is the most reliable monitor. A stethoscope-audible air embolism is a large one. Retrieval of the embolism through a central line is described but is not the first line management of the condition. Immediate action involves resuscitation, 100% oxygen, flooding the wound site with saline and elevating central venous pressure by applying the head-down position and compressing the neck veins.

Ref: Clinical Neuroanaesthesia, Churchill Livingstone 1990.

ANSWER   64

A. TRUE   B. FALSE   C. FALSE   D. TRUE   E. TRUE

Increased plasma levels whilst standing are due to a decrease in the rate of removal by the liver and a postural increase in renin secretion which stimulates aldosterone release. Primary hyperaldosteronism (Conn's syndrome) occurs with aldosterone secreting tumours of the adrenal cortex. Na reabsorption is achieved by K or H exchange in the distal tubule.

Ref: Ganong WF. Review of Medical Physiology. Lange., Ch20

ANSWER   65

A. TRUE   B. TRUE   C. TRUE   D. FALSE   E. TRUE

Local anaesthetics are poorly effective in areas of ambient acidity such as around dental abscesses, and so general anaesthesia is sometimes indicated in these situations. Children with Down's syndrome often have cardiac anomalies in which case prophylactic antibiotics are necessary. Inpatient dental surgery usually involves more complex work than outpatient surgery, and nasal intubation with insertion of a pack is usual - although more people are using the laryngeal mask airway for this purpose. The maxillary nerve is the second division of the trigeminal. Tachycardia and hypertension are seen with high concentrations of a vaso-pressor to local anaesthetics used in dental surgery where absorption from the mucosa is rapid.

ANSWER   66

A. TRUE   B. TRUE   C. TRUE   D. TRUE   E. FALSE

Simple humidifiers consist of a water bath that is often heated. This bath has been a common site for pseudomonas infection in the ITU setting. Attempts to reduce the risk of pseudomonal colonisation include heating the water in the bath to 60°C, however this runs the risk of the inspired gases scalding the patient. With heated baths the water vapour tends to condense out in the tubing as it cools on its way to the patient. Without water-traps there is a risk of puddles of water obstructing the tubing. The HME can also be obstructed if it becomes filled with secretions from the endotracheal tube. Ultrasonic nebulisers are very efficient humidifiers capable of producing a relative humidity of 200% at 37.°C. In babies particularly this can quickly lead to water overload. Reduction of heat loss is said to be one of the benefits of humidification.

Ref: Davis PD, Parbrook GD, Kenny GNC. Basic Physics and Measurement in Anaesthesia, 4th edn. Butterworth-Heinemann, 1995

ANSWER 67

A. TRUE   B. TRUE   C. TRUE   D. TRUE   E. FALSE

Oxygen can be measured by paramagnetic and electrochemical techniques as well as by Raman scattering and mass spectrometry. Electrochemical techniques including the galvanic (or fuel) cell and the polarographic (Clark) electrode. Ultra-violet absorption spectroscopy has been used to measure halothane concentration.

Ref: Dorsch JA, Dorsch SE. Understanding Anesthesia Equipment; Construction, Care and Complications, 2nd edn. Williams & Wilkins, 1984

ANSWER 68

A. FALSE   B. TRUE   C. TRUE   D. TRUE   E. TRUE

Confidence intervals are the range of values derived from sample data relating the data to the actual population. 95% confidence intervals contain the true (population) value with a probability (p value) of 0.05. This corresponds to +/-1.96 standard error of the means (SEM) from the reference value. Confidence intervals are preferred because they indicate the likely magnitude of differences between sample values by giving a range within which the true value lies. By using the same unit as the data, they allow estimations of clinical relevance to be made; for example, a statistically very significant result may be clinically irrelevant if the actual differences involved are small.

Ref: Yentis, Hirsch, Smith. Anaesthesia A to Z. Butterworth-Heinemann

ANSWER 69

A. TRUE   B. TRUE   C. FALSE   D. TRUE   E. FALSE

Prolactin promotes breast development and milk formation during pregnancy. It stimulates release of dopamine in the hypothalamus which in turn inhibits the release of FSH, LHRH and further prolactin. Secretion of prolactin is stimulated by TRH resulting in excessive levels of prolactin in hypothyroidism. The sucking stimulus via the maternal mamilla is the signal for a very high production of prolactin during lactation. Stress and drugs (morphine, reserpine, phenothiazines) inhibit dopamine release, facilitating prolactin release.

Ref: Despopoulos A, Silbernagl S. Color Atlas of Physiology, 232-271

ANSWER 70

A. FALSE   B. FALSE   C. FALSE   D. FALSE   E. TRUE

There are two patterns of sleep. NREM sleep which is divided into four stages and makes up 75% of total sleep time. REM sleep is associated with rapid low-amplitude irregular EEG activity, dreaming, a reduction in skeletal muscle tone, tachypnoea, tachycardia, penile erection and dreaming.

Ref: Yentis, Hirsch, Smith. Anaesthesia A to Z. Butterworth-Heinemann

ANSWER 71

A. TRUE   B. TRUE   C. FALSE   D. FALSE   E. TRUE

70% of HCO_3 formed in the RBC diffuses into the plasma and is balanced by an inward chloride ion shift that increases intracellular osmolality. Deoxygenated Hb buffers the rising hydrogen ion concentration in the RBC allowing further HCO_3 formation (Haldane effect). Plasma proteins may form carbamino bonds with CO_2.

Ref: Despopoulos A, Silbernagl S. Color Atlas of Physiology. 78-108.

ANSWER 72

A. TRUE   **B. FALSE**   **C. TRUE**   **D. FALSE**   **E. TRUE**

It irreversibly acetylates cyclo-oxygenase. Higher doses affect vessel wall enzymes resulting in reductions in PGI_2 production. It may inhibit platelet function for up to 10 days following cessation of therapy during which time new platelets are generated.

ANSWER 73

A. FALSE   **B. TRUE**   **C. TRUE**   **D. TRUE**   **E. TRUE**

Nociception is associated with free nerve endings, whereas specialised nerve endings have been identified for particular sensory modalities, eg. Meissners corpuscles (touch), Pacinian corpuscles (vibration and proprioception), Ruffini corpuscles (proprioception).

Ref: Yentis, Hirsch, Smith. Anaesthesia A to Z. Butterworth-Heinemann

ANSWER 74

A. TRUE   **B. FALSE**   **C. FALSE**   **D. TRUE**   **E. TRUE**

The three methods of measuring FRC are plethysmography, nitrogen wash-out and helium wash-in. Spirometry will measure all lung volumes except FRC, residual volume and TLC. Intra-oesophageal balloons are used to measure intra-pleural pressure.

Ref: Nunn JF. Applied Respiratory Physiology. Butterworth-Heinemann

ANSWER 75

A. FALSE   **B. FALSE**   **C. FALSE**   **D. TRUE**   **E. TRUE**

Hypokalaemia causes P-R prolongation, ST depression, T wave inversion and prominent U waves.

Ref: Ganong WF. Review of Medical Physiology. Lange.

ANSWER 76

A. TRUE   **B. FALSE**   **C. FALSE**   **D. TRUE**   **E. FALSE**

For sterilisation or disinfection to be effective decontamination must precede them. Pressurised steam is commonly used for sterilisation, but low pressure low temperature (74°C) steam may be used for disinfection, and for sterilisation with the addition of formaldehyde vapour. Dry heat (at 150-170°C) is useful for sterilising some items. Pasteurisation is a form of disinfection.

Ref: Davey A, Moyle JTB, Ward CS. Ward's Anaesthetic Equipment, 3rd edn. W.B. Saunders, 1992

ANSWER 77

A. TRUE   **B. TRUE**   **C. FALSE**   **D. FALSE**   **E. TRUE**

Progesterone is thermogenic and probably accounts for the rise in basal temperature that accompanies ovulation in the normal menstrual cycle. It stimulates respiration via a central effect, delays gastric emptying and causes vascular smooth muscle relaxation and hence reduces SVR. Post-delivery progesterone returns to non-pregnant levels within 24 hours.

Ref: Ganong W F. Review of Medical Physiology. Lange. Yentis, Hirsch, Smith. Anaesthesia A to Z. Butterworth-Heinemann.

ANSWER 78
A. TRUE B. FALSE C. TRUE D. FALSE E. TRUE

Tachyphylaxis is acute tolerance. Positive co-operativity is likely to occur when multiple sites within a tightly coupled group of receptors must be occupied in order to initiate an event (eg Ach opening a postjunctional ion channel at the NMJ, and the action of non-depolarizing relaxants in blocking that event).

Plasma concentration = Mass of drug injected / Apparent volume of distribution

If the drug is highly lipid soluble plasma concentration will be low resulting in an apparently large volume of distribution.

Ref: Nunn, Utting, Brown. General Anaesthesia. Butterworths.

ANSWER 79
A. FALSE B. TRUE C. TRUE D. FALSE E. TRUE

The anion gap reflects metabolic, not respiratory, acidosis and although it may be elevated for other reasons (e.g. sepsis) is not a universal finding. Respiratory failure represents an imbalance between supply and demand, although it is usually a deficiency on the supply side rather than an increase in oxygen requirement. Oxygen administration will improve V/Q mismatch but does little to improve shunt due to the shape of the oxygen dissociation curve.

Ref: Nunn, Utting, Burnell Brown. General Anaesthesia. Butterworth-Heinemann

ANSWER 80
A. TRUE B. FALSE C. FALSE D. TRUE E. TRUE

Ketamine hydrochloride (a phencyclidine derivative) is presented as a racaemic mixture. The isomers have different pharmacological properties but similar kinetics, suggesting the presence of specific receptors. The S isomer is about 2 times more potent as the racemic mixture and 4 times more potent than the R isomer. Recovery is also faster with the S isomer. Ketamine is not significantly protein bound but is highly lipid soluble. It is metabolised in the liver and one of the metabolites (norketamine) is active with a potency of around 30 % of the parent drug.

PHYSICAL:
 pH 3.5-5.5, pKa 7.5, 12% albumin bound

DOSE:
 1-2 mg/kg iv, 10 mg/kg im

Ref: Nimmo, Rowbotham, Smith. Anaesthesia. Blackwell

ANSWER 81
A. TRUE B. FALSE C. FALSE D. TRUE E. FALSE

A sample is taken from a population. A population is a group who share a parameter, for example, being male, bald or surgical patients. The mean is the arithmetical average, the median the measurement which is exactly mid way between the ends of all the measurements ranked in order, and the mode is the most commonly observed measurement.

ANSWER 82

A. FALSE   B. TRUE   C. TRUE   D. TRUE   E. TRUE

Propofol is highly protein bound (97%). It has a volume of distribution at steady state of about 1000 litres. It is presented as an emulsion containing an isotonic 1% solution. Metabolism is in the liver with about 40% undergoing conjugation to a glucoronide and 60% metabolised to a quinol which is excreted as a glucoronide and sulphate. The metabolic clearance exceeds hepatic blood flow, suggesting extra-hepatic sites of metabolism. Only about 0.3% is excreted unchanged. A quinol metabolite is responsible for the discolouration of urine. It is safe in both MH and porphyria. About 15% of patients develop excitatory movements on induction. A fat overload syndrome, with hyperlipidaemia, and fatty infiltration of heart, liver, kidneys and lungs can follow prolonged infusion.

Ref: Nimmo, Rowbotham, Smith: Anaesthesia: chapter 6

ANSWER 83

A. TRUE   B. FALSE   C. FALSE   D. FALSE   E. TRUE

ABO compatible blood is fully compatible in 97% cases, 98% if Rh compatible. Rh negative = Absence of C,D & E antigens. Those of group AB (3% of population) have serum free of anti-A or anti-B Abs. Rhesus incompatible cells are bound by IgG antbodies that do not activate complement.

Ref: Cotreras M. ABC of Transfusion. BMJ Publications, 1994

ANSWER 84

A. TRUE   B. TRUE   C. TRUE   D. FALSE   E. FALSE

Amiodarone can cause both hypo- and hyperthyroidism. Hypotension and atrio-ventricular block have been reported after intravenous injection. Pulmonary effects include diffuse alveolitis and fibrosis. Other side effects include corneal microdeposits, CNS toxicity, cirrhosis and gastrointestinal upset. Photosensitivity can be a· major problem. Lupus-like syndromes are associated with procainamide and hydralazine.

ANSWER 85

A. TRUE   B. TRUE   C. FALSE   D. TRUE   E. FALSE

The rate-limiting step is passage across the stratum corneum of the skin. Uptake depends on the physico-chemical properties of the agent and delivery system. Although they have similar molecular weights, fentanyl is less water soluble and more lipid soluble than morphine, and has a skin flux some 160 times greater than morphine. Hyoscine, fentanyl and GTN are the commonly used transdermal delivery systems in anaesthesia.

ANSWER 86

A. TRUE   B. TRUE   C. FALSE   D. TRUE   E. FALSE

Hepatic bile is produced continuously and is stored and concentrated in the gall bladder where it becomes more viscous.

Ref:·Despopoulos A, Silbernagl S. Color Atlas of Physiology, 196-231

ANSWER 87

A. FALSE   B. TRUE   C. FALSE   D. TRUE   E. FALSE

Factors which increase flow out of capillaries are increased capillary hydrostatic pressure, increased interstitial colloid osmotic pressure, reduced interstitial hydrostatic pressure or reduced colloid osmotic pressure. In certain conditions (eg sepsis) the permeability coefficient may be altered.

Ref: Ganong WF. Review of Medical Physiology. Lange. Ch1.

ANSWER 88

A. FALSE   B. TRUE   C. TRUE   D. FALSE   E. TRUE

The vitamin K dependent factors are II (Prothrombin), VII, IX & X. Normally vitamin K is provided by intestinal bacteria, but if the gut flora has been wiped out deficiency may occur. A, D, E & K are fat-soluble and dependent upon normal fat absorption. Contact between factor XII & collagen fibres triggers the intrinsic pathway. Antithrombin 3 is the most important plasma protein involved in protection against thrombosis. It forms complexes with thrombin & factor Xa preventing further activity. Heparin promotes its activity.

Ref: Despopoulos A, Silbernagl S. Color Atlas of Physiology, 60-77

ANSWER 89

A. FALSE   B. TRUE   C. FALSE   D. TRUE   E. TRUE

The coroner need not be informed of a postoperative death if the cause is established, although it is often wise to discuss a postop death with him or his representative before, for example, signing a cremation certificate. Neither is it necessary if the patient was seen within 14 days, again, so long as the cause is established. The list of reasons to report includes: sudden death not seen by doctor within 14 days, murder, suicide, drugs, poisons and as a result of medical treatment; industrial accident; patient in receipt of a pension, whether industrial, disability or war; alcohol, self neglect; death of an infant or of a foster child; following abortion; in custody or prison; and as a result of a road traffic accident.

ANSWER 90

A. TRUE   B. TRUE   C. FALSE   D. TRUE   E.FALSE

Pulse pressure is the difference between systolic and diastolic pressure, usually ~ 40 mmHg. It is increased by increased stroke volume, reduced compliance of the arterial tree (eg elderly) and if measured peripherally in the arterial tree.

Ref: Yentis, Hirsch, Smith. Anaesthesia A to Z. Butterworth-Heinemann

NOTES

NOTES

NOTES

QBase Anaesthesia
on CD-ROM

SYSTEM REQUIREMENTS

An IBM compatible PC with a minimum 80386 processor and 4Mb of RAM

VGA Monitor set up to display at least 256 colours

CD-ROM drive

Windows 3.1 or higher with Microsoft compatible mouse

INSTALLATION INSTRUCTIONS

The program will install the appropriate files onto your hard drive. It requires the QBase CD-ROM to be installed in the D:\drive.

In order to run QBase the CD-ROM must be in the drive.

Print Readme.txt and Helpfile.txt on the CD-ROM for fuller instructions and user manual

WINDOWS 95

1. Insert the QBase CD-ROM into the drive **D:**

2. From the **Start Menu,** select the RUN **option**

3. Type **D:\setup.exe and press enter or return**

4. **Follow the Full Installation** option and accept the default directory for installation of QBase.

   The installation program creates a folder called **QBase** containing the program icon and another called **Exams** into which you can save previous exam attempts.

5. To run QBase double click the **QBase** icon in the QBase folder. From Windows Explorer double click the **QBase.exe** file in the QBase folder.

WINDOWS 3.1/WINDOWS FOR WORKGROUPS 3.11

1. Insert the QBase CD-ROM into the drive **D:**

2. From the **File Menu,** select the **RUN option**

3. Type **D:\setup.exe and press enter or return**

4. Follow the instructions given by the installation program. Select the **Full Installation** option and accept the default directory for installation of QBase

   The installation program creates a program window and directory called **QBase** containing the program icon. It also creates a directory called **Exams** into which you can save previous attempts.

5. To run QBase double click on the **QBase** icon in the QBase program. From File Manager double click the **QBase.exe** file in the QBase directory